Laboratory Diagnosis of Fungal Infections:

A Manual for Processing Specimens, Microscopy and Culture Techniques

By:

Mohamed E. Hamid
Martin R.P. Joseph
Mohammed M. Assiry

17.78 x 25.4 cm
Color on White paper, 82 pages

Copyright ©2014, M.E. Hamid, M.R.P. Joseph, M.M. Assiry
ISBN-13: 978-1492314028
ISBN-10: 1492314021

All rights reserved

Printed By:
CreateSpace: A DBA of On-Demand Publishing LLC, part of the Amazon group of companies

((Most hospitals do not perform mycologic examinations because laboratory personnel still believe in the "old wive's tale" that mycology is too difficult to do and that the fungi are too infectious to handle...... It is hoped that laboratories will take the initiative in offering diagnostic mycology services routinely. Medical mycology can be both a challenge and a rewarding experience to those who choose to become involved))

G.D. Roberts (Human Pathology, 1976, 7, pp. 161-168)

TABLE OF CONTENTS

Page

PREFACE	5
ACKNOWLEDGEMENTS	6
HOW TO USE THE MANUAL?	7
FUNGI: INTRODUCTORY REMARKS	8
SECTION ONE: GENERAL APPROACH TO THE DIAGNOSIS OF SUSPECTED FUNGAL INFECTION	10
Diagnosis of suspected fungal infections: An Overview	11
Safety precautions and handling of specimens	12
Direct microscopy	14
Culture	15
indirect microscopy	16
Histopathology	17
SECTION TWO: COLLECTION, PROCESSING, MICROSCOPY AND CULTURE OF CLINICAL SPECIMENS	21
Skin, hair and nails	22
Sputum and other respiratory specimens	23
Tissue biopsy	24
Blood and bone marrow	25
CSF and brain abscess aspirate	26
Pus, exudates, grains and drainage	27
Vaginal swab and discharge	28
Urine	29
SECTION THREE: SCHEMES FOR FUNGAL IDENTIFICATION	30
Yeasts	32
Dematiaceous molds	35
Hyaline molds	40
Dimorphic fungi	54
SECTION FOUR: A SUMMARY TABLE	58
Specimen collection, fungal stains, cultures and commonly isolated fungi from different body sites	59
SECTION FIVE: CULTURE MEDIA, STAINS AND MICROSCOPIC TECHNIQUES	64
Culture media	65
Sabouraud Dextrose Agar (SDA)	65
Sabouraud Dextrose Agar with antibiotics	65
Brain Heart Infusion broth (BHIB)	66
Brain Heart Infusion Agar (BHIA) with 5% Sheep Blood	67
BHIA with 5% Sheep Blood and antibiotics	67
Dermatophyte Test Medium (DTM)	68
Stains	69

    10% Potassium Hydroxide (KOH) 69
    10% Potassium Hydroxide (KOH) with Parker Ink 69
    Lactophenol Cotton Blue (LPCB) 70
    India ink 70
    Calcofluor White with 10% KOH 71
    Gram's stain 72
    Grocott's Methenamine Silver (GMS) stain 72
    Periodic acid-Schiff (PAS) 73
    Giemsa's stain 74
Microscopic techniques 75
    Tease mount technique 75
    Cellotape Flag Preparations 75
    Micro culture (Slide Culture) technique 77

REFERENCES 78

INDEX 79

PREFACE

Diseases caused by fungi are steadily increasing and have become significant medical problems. The number of fungal species isolated from patients suffering from various diseases is increasing as well, some of these species had previously been considered harmless. The increases in the number of immune-deficient patients, beside the greater understanding and awareness of opportunistic fungal infections, have drawn attention to the importance of early and accurate detection of fungi in clinical specimens.

This manual describes briefly how to make a laboratory diagnosis of suspected fungal diseases. The diagnosis begins after receiving a good quality clinical specimen, then how to process it and or store it, taking into account basic safety procedures. Subsequently, the manual explains the diagnostic process step by step using schematic charts and a number of macroscopic and microscopic illustrations and pictures

Many microbiology or mycology books list topics according to names of diseases or names or types of fungi. However, this book chooses the clinical specimens as the main topic and describes how "good quality" specimens are collected, stored, and transported before laboratory processing. It describes the major laboratory steps *(direct microscopy, culture, indirect microscopy and histopathology)*. These tests take aliquots from the original specimens and then each test establishes the diagnosis either alone or in integration with other tests and considering the clinical diagnosis provided with the request form. Therefore, a diagnostic microbiology laboratory does all tests or selects some according to facilities, experience and need. For those reasons, the appropriate collection and transportation of clinical specimens represents a key step towards establishing a confirmation to the clinical diagnosis. The routine identification of fungi depends mainly on the morphological examination of microscopic structures, particularly spores and conidia, as well as the specialized cells that produce them. Therefore, we recommend and we have applied these methods considerably.

As a short handbook, this effort enables practitioners, laboratory technicians and researchers to accomplish laboratory diagnosis and identification of unknown fungus to the *Genus* level. However, we have explained methods to reaching identification to species levels to some important fungal groups namely: dermatophytes, *Candida* and *Aspergillus* species. Details for species identification can be found elsewhere. When you know the genus or you have doubts between two or three genera, then you can find details in many textbooks and web sites. For this purpose we have provided references and websites at the end of the book.

Mohamed E. Hamid	***Martin R.P. Joseph***	***M.Mushabab Assiry***
(BVSc, MSc, PhD, AvH Fellow)	*(BSc, MSc, PhD)*	*(BSc)*
Department of Microbiology,	*Department of Microbiology,*	*The Laboratories,*
College of Medicine, King Khalid	*College of Medicine, King*	*Aseer Central Hospital*
University, Abha, KSA	*Khalid University, Abha, KSA*	*Abha, KSA*

ACKNOWLEDGEMENTS

Most of the macroscopic and microscopic pictures of various fungi used in this manual have been jointly diagnosed at the Microbiology Laboratory, Aseer Central Hospital and the Department of Microbiology, College of Medicine, King Khalid University (Abha). **Pictures** and illustrations **cited from other sources** have been acknowledged, as appropriate, throughout the pages of this book

The authors thank the staff of the Microbiology Laboratories especially Dr Faten Al Abd and Mr Waleed Haimor, Aseer Central Hospital and the Department of Microbiology, College of Medicine, King Khalid University for facilitating the use of materials and amenities that enabled us to complete this project.

HOW TO USE THE MANUAL?

AT A GLANCE
All steps for making lab. diagnosis are summarized in **SECTION ONE**

IF YOU RECEIVE A SPECIMEN
Follow instructions and methods for each type of specimens; one page in **SECTION TWO**

IF YOU HAVE A HISTOPATHOLOGY SECTION
Record what you found e.g. Grains; then compare it with models in **SECTION ONE**

WHEN YOU GOT FUNGAL GRWOTH
Follow Identification Charts **SECTION THREE**
Establish the type of fungus (broad group): Yeast, Hyaline mold or a Dematiaceous mold. Submit report to doctors giving the Genus name
Then go to next step down

MAKE FULL IDENTIFICATION
Follow Identification Charts (e.g. a yeast growh; then go to yeast pages in the Identification Charts **SECTION THREE** to establishing Genus and Species if you can, if not consult one of the references for details description of genera and species… in **REFERENCE SECTION**

TECHNIQUES AND METHODS
Details of culture media, staining and summary of specimens and what to do with them are available in **SECTION FIVE**

FUNGI: INTRODUCTORY REMARKS

- Definitions:
    - A fungus (pl. fungi) is a member of a large group of eukaryotic organisms that includes microorganisms such as yeasts and molds (moulds), as well as mushrooms
    - Mycology: The study of fungi
    - Mycoses: fungal diseases
    - Mycotoxins: fungal toxins

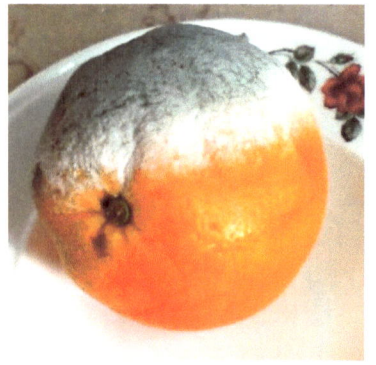 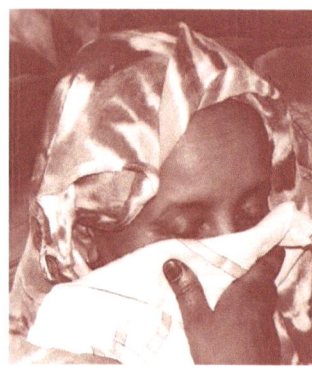 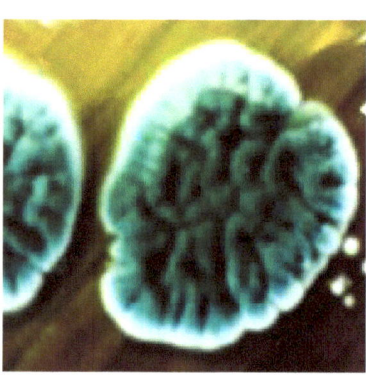

Fungi are everywhere! With a wide host range   Allergy from molds   *Penicillium* species: a source for beta lactam antibiotics

- Characteristics:
    - Plant like eukaryotes but no chlorophyll
    - Widely distributed in nature both useful and causes of diseases
    - Most are multicellular (molds), but some are unicellular (yeasts)
    - Cell walls: contains high chitin (a complex polysaccharide)
    - Cell membrane: contains high sterols (target for antifungals)
    - Non-motile and chemoheterotrophic (= getting energy from organic molecules)
    - Grow as hyphae; hyphal networks are called mycelium
- Reproduction
    - Asexual: *Budding, Sporulation, Fragmentation*
    - Sexual: *Meiosis, Zygospore formation*
- Ecology
    - Fungi are often inconspicuous, occur in every environment on earth
    - Play important roles in most ecosystems. Along with bacteria, fungi are the major decomposers in most terrestrial (and some aquatic) ecosystems
    - Symbiosis: Many fungi have important symbiotic relationships with organisms from most if not all Kingdoms, e.g. *Mycorrhizae* (fungus with plant roots) Lichens (fungus with algae)

- Importance of fungi
    - Decomposers and recyclers of nutrients
    - Yeasts are used to make beer & bread
    - Help form blue cheeses
    - Citric acid in Coke is produced by *Aspergillus niger*
    - *Aspergillus* is used to make soy sauce
    - Some are edible (Mushrooms)
    - Beta-lactam antibiotics such as penicillins are produced by *Penicillium* molds
    - Some are internal or external parasites (cause diseases)
    - Some fungi are poisonous: e.g. *Amanita* mushroom
    - Fungal spores cause allergies
    - Damage crops: molds, mildew, rusts & smuts
- Classification

    Many types of classification are available, but for simplicity we are adopting the morphological one. On this basis fungi are divided into:

    1. Yeasts
    2. Molds [mold (US) or mould (UK)]
        a. Hyaline molds
        b. Dematiaceous (pigmented) molds
    3. Dimorphic fungi

SECTION ONE: GENERAL APPROACH TO THE DIAGNOSIS OF SUSPECTED FUNGAL INFECTION

DIAGNOSIS OF SUSPECTED FUNGAL INFECTIONS: AN OVERVIEW

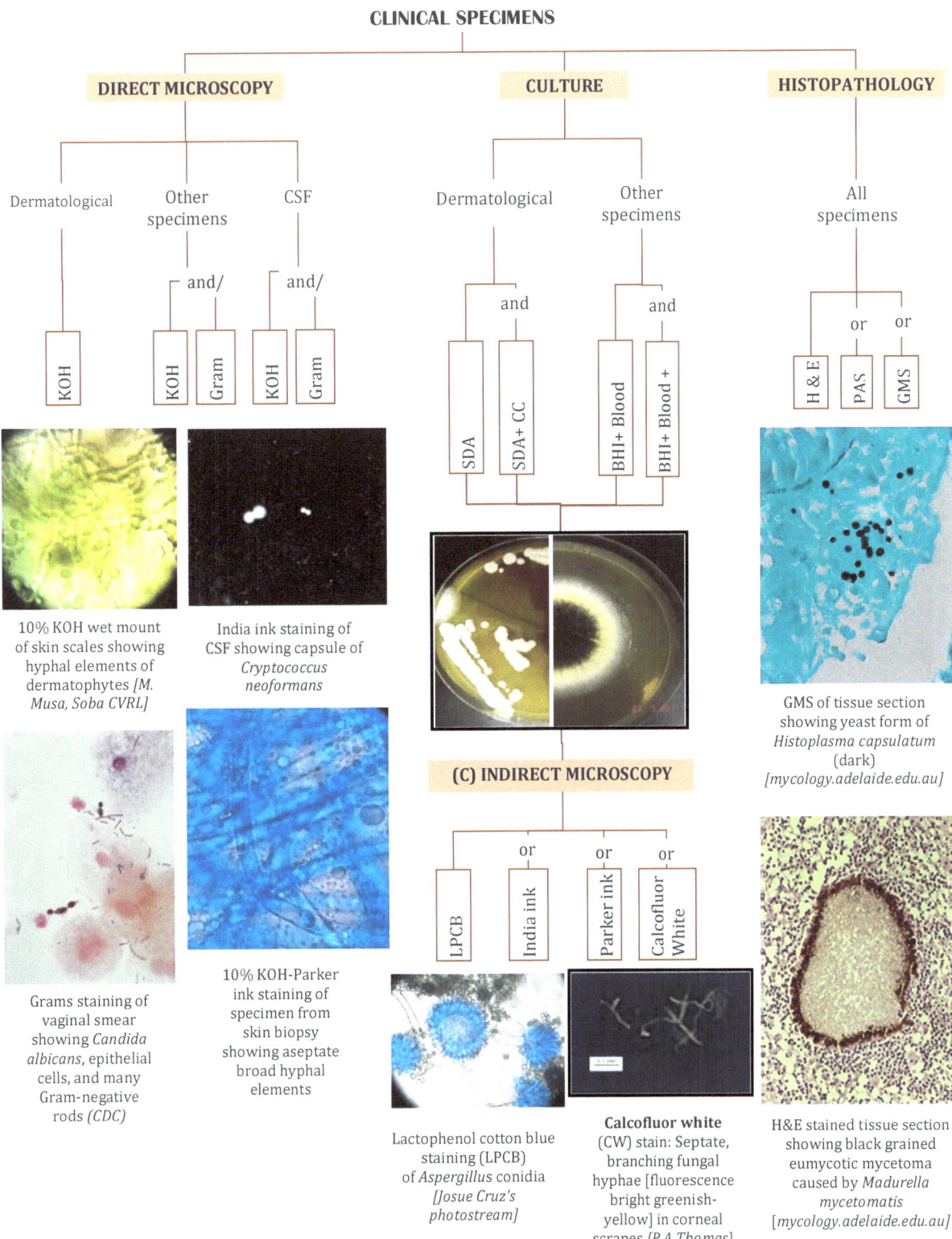

* Abbreviations and details of stains and media are given in Section Five

SAFETY PRECAUTIONS AND HANDLING OF SPECIMENS

Gloves and coats
- Wear laboratory coat, gloves and a mask when handling clinical specimens and when working with fungal culture

BSC
Work on a BSC (Biological Safety Cabinet) level 2 or 3 (hazard of fungal spores)

Aseptic technique
- Collect specimens aseptically

Containers
- Use sterile containers (wide-mouthed, plastic with a screw-on lid, and leak-proof)

Labeling
- Label and date the container appropriately and complete the requisition form

Biohazard bag
- Transport specimen to the lab in a biohazard bag should be secured and labeled "**Biohazard**"

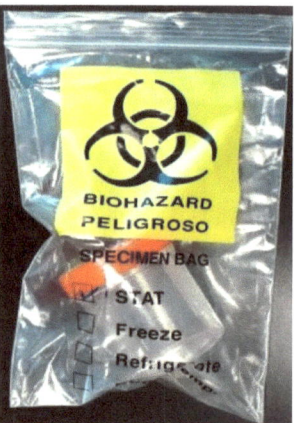

Delivery
- Deliver specimens to the lab within 2 hours of collection since overgrowth by contaminating bacteria and/or saprophytic fungi is common

Storage: If transport is delayed, store:
- Blood, bone marrow and CSF at body temperature (**30 ºC -37 ºC**)
- Dermatological specimens at room temperature (**25 ºC**)
- Other specimens at refrigerator **(4 ºC)**

Spills
- Work areas and surfaces should be disinfected daily with 1% sodium hypochlorite (household bleach). Use 10% bleach to clean up spills after wiping the surface clean
- Contaminated non-disposable equipment should be soaked in 1% household bleach for 5 minutes. Before use wash in soapy water and sterilize if necessary. Heavily soiled disposable items should be soaked in 10% household bleach before incineration or disposal

Cleaning and washing

- Clean your **bench** area with a disinfectant: Phenols (e.g. Lysol 1-5%) or Halogens (e.g. 0.1-5% Ca or Na hypochlorite)

- **Wash your hands** before leaving

Rejection

Causes for rejection of clinical specimens

1. **Unlabeled** specimen
2. Insufficient **quantity** (empty swab)
3. **Contamination** suspected
4. **Haemolysed** blood sample
5. Specimen submitted in **syringe with needle** attached
6. Inappropriate **transport or storage**
7. Unknown time **delay** (usually more than 72 hours)
8. Specimen received after **leaking** transport container into specimen bag

DIRECT MICROSCOPY

Dermatological
[Hair, nails, and scrapings]

CNS
[CSF]

Other specimens
[Respiratory, pus, biopsy, blood, fluid,

KOH mount *[Hair, nails, and skin scrapings]*
- In a clean slide place a drop of 10% KOH-Parker ink [*prepared by dissolving 10g KOH in 80 ml DW, add 10 ml glycerol and 10 ml Parker ink*] (**use 40% for nails**)
- Using inoculating needle, place small portion of specimen in the KOH drop
- Place a cover slide and squash gently
- Blot off excess fluid
- Gently heat by passing 2-4 times through flame [don't boil]to allow digestion of specimen
- Wait 20 min [several hours for nails] *Apply fingernail at margin of cover slide to prevent dryness of slide*
- Examine microscopically for faintly blue stained fungal elements
- Negative specimen should be kept and re-examined after 1 hour or next day

(Digestion of skin sample can be done in small tube then one drop is transferred to slide, 1-2 drops of LPCB or Parker ink added, mixed, cover slide place and examined)

India ink *[CSF]*
- place a loopful of India ink on a clean slide
- mix
- Place a clean cover slip over the preparation avoiding air bubbles
- press down, or blot gently with a filter paper strip to get a thin, even film
- Examine under dry objectives followed by oil immersion

Gram
- Make a thin smear, fix by heat
- Flood with Gram's crystal violet for 1 min, then rinse with water
- Stain with Gram's iodine (a mordant) for 1 min, rinse again
- Decolorize with Gram decolorizes (95% alcohol) for 20 seconds, and Rinse
- Counter stain with Safranin red solution for 1 min, Rinse
- Carefully blot the slide dry with bibulous paper and Observe under the microscope
- Gram +ve stain purple; Gram –ve stain red

KOH
- Place a small portion of specimen in a drop of 10% KOH
- (details in dermatological (left)

Mold hyphae, yeast cells

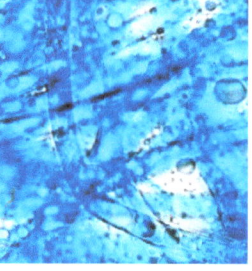

10% KOH-Parker ink staining of pus showing hyphal elements of a zygomycete

Yeast cells with capsules of budding

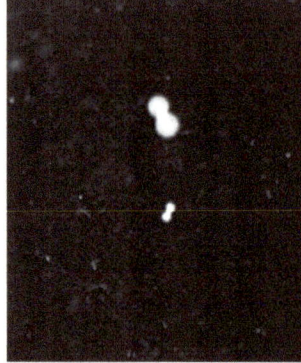

India ink staining of CSF showing capsule of *Cryptococcus neoformans*

Yeast cells, Bacteria, Spores of molds

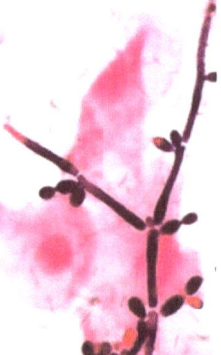

Grams staining of vaginal smear showing *C. albicans*, epithelial cells, and many Gram-negative rods (*Dan Wiedbrauk*)

Mold hyphae and Yeast cells

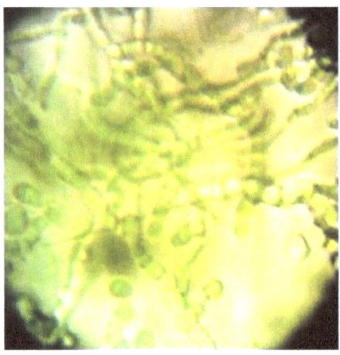

10% KOH of skin scales showing arthrospores (broken hyphae) of *Trichophyton* sp. *(Moh Musa. Soba. Sudan)*

CULTURE

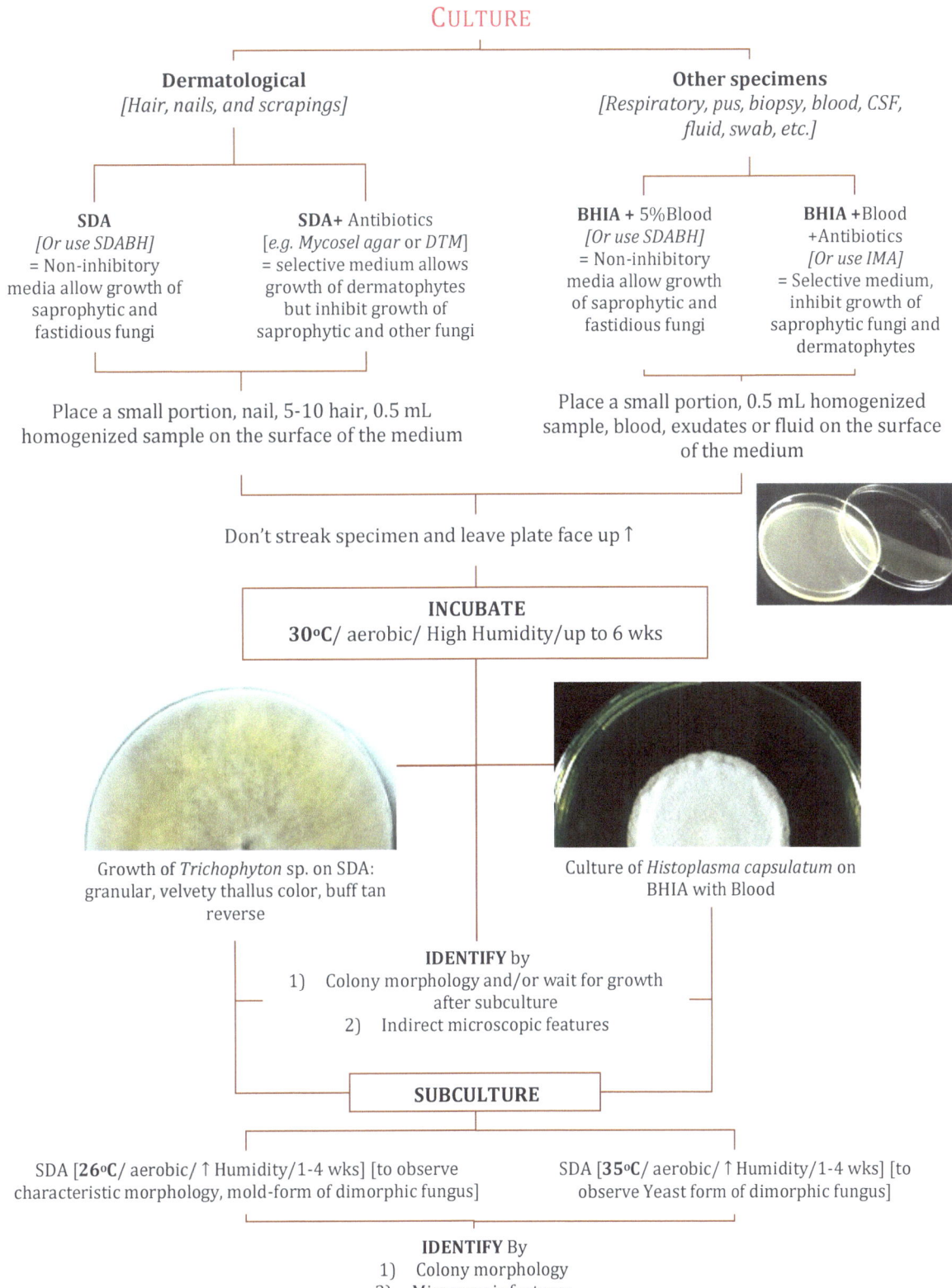

Dermatological
[Hair, nails, and scrapings]

- **SDA**
  [Or use SDABH]
  = Non-inhibitory media allow growth of saprophytic and fastidious fungi

- **SDA+ Antibiotics**
  [e.g. Mycosel agar or DTM]
  = selective medium allows growth of dermatophytes but inhibit growth of saprophytic and other fungi

Place a small portion, nail, 5-10 hair, 0.5 mL homogenized sample on the surface of the medium

Other specimens
[Respiratory, pus, biopsy, blood, CSF, fluid, swab, etc.]

- **BHIA + 5%Blood**
  [Or use SDABH]
  = Non-inhibitory media allow growth of saprophytic and fastidious fungi

- **BHIA +Blood +Antibiotics**
  [Or use IMA]
  = Selective medium, inhibit growth of saprophytic fungi and dermatophytes

Place a small portion, 0.5 mL homogenized sample, blood, exudates or fluid on the surface of the medium

Don't streak specimen and leave plate face up ↑

INCUBATE
30°C/ aerobic/ High Humidity/up to 6 wks

Growth of *Trichophyton* sp. on SDA: granular, velvety thallus color, buff tan reverse

Culture of *Histoplasma capsulatum* on BHIA with Blood

IDENTIFY by
1) Colony morphology and/or wait for growth after subculture
2) Indirect microscopic features

SUBCULTURE

SDA [26°C/ aerobic/ ↑ Humidity/1-4 wks] [to observe characteristic morphology, mold-form of dimorphic fungus]

SDA [35°C/ aerobic/ ↑ Humidity/1-4 wks] [to observe Yeast form of dimorphic fungus]

IDENTIFY By
1) Colony morphology
2) Microscopic features

*Abbreviations and details of stains and media are given in Section Five

INDIRECT MICROSCOPY

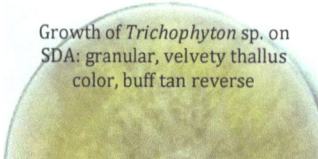

Growth of *Trichophyton* sp. on SDA: granular, velvety thallus color, buff tan reverse

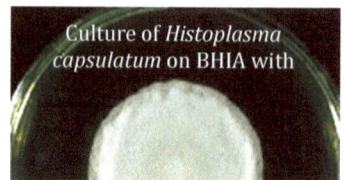

Culture of *Histoplasma capsulatum* on BHIA with

Smear or mount for microscopy can be prepared by one of the e following methods:

Tease mount technique
- Wear gloves and work in a BSC
- Pick small portion of colony with its underlying agar using a dissecting needle
- Place it on a drop of LPCB on a clean slide [*placed slide on top of an inverted Petri dish*]
- Tease gently the colony apart with the dissecting needle
- Overlay [cover] with coverslip
- Apply gentle pressure using the eraser of a pencil to make an even mount
- Examine fungal elements with 10X then 40X then 100X
- *Advantage: Easy to use*
- *Disadvantage: Disturbs the delicate fruiting fungal structure and spores*

Cellotape technique
- Wear gloves and work in a BSC
- Cut a 2 cm x 2 cm piece of a clear cellotape [*can use a flag by sticking one of its end to a wooden stick*]
- Press gently the sticky side of the tape onto the colony surface
- Place the tape onto a slide containing drop of LPCB or Aniline Blue [*placed slide on top of an inverted Petri dish*]
- Blot off excess stain and stick ends of tape to the slide
- Examine fungal elements with 10X then 40X then 100X
- *Advantage: Easy to use and may not disturb fungal microscopic morphology*
- *Disadvantage: BSC required spores*

Microculture technique
- Wear gloves and work in a BSC
- Place a piece of filter paper or gauze on the bottom of a sterile Petri dish
- Place sterile rods or sticks on top of the filter paper
- Place slide on the rods
- Place a block of agar [*potato or cornmeal agar*] on top of the slide [*round block made by tube can be used*]
- Inoculate the margins of the agar block from the culture to be examined
- heat a coverslip and immediately place it on top of the agar block
- Pipette water to the bottom of the plate
- Place the lid of the Petri dish and incubate at 30°C/ 3-5 days
- when growth appears, gently remove the coverslip and place it on to of slide containing 2 drops of LPCB
- Use fingernail to seal the coverslip on the slide for prolong use
- Examine fungal elements with 10X then 40X then 100X
- *Advantage: fungal structure can be seen clearly*
- *Disadvantage: takes time and need special care spores*

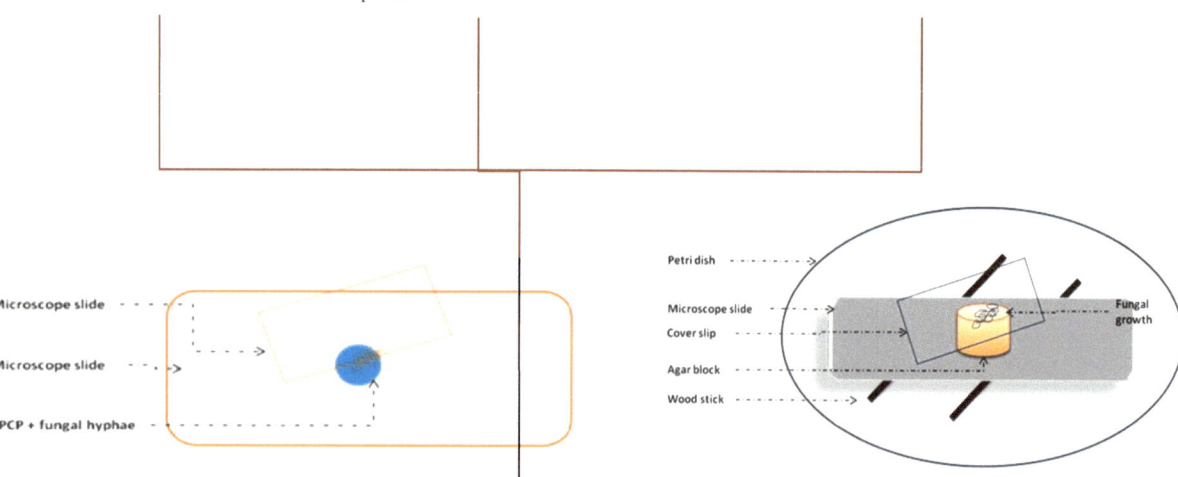

IDENTIFY By
- Colony morphology
- Microscopic features

HISTOPATHOLOGY

Haematoxylin and Eosin (H &E) | Periodic Acid-Schiff (PAS) | Gomori methenamine silver (GMS) | Giemsa stain (Useful in aspirates)

PRESENCE OF BUDDING YEAST CELLS

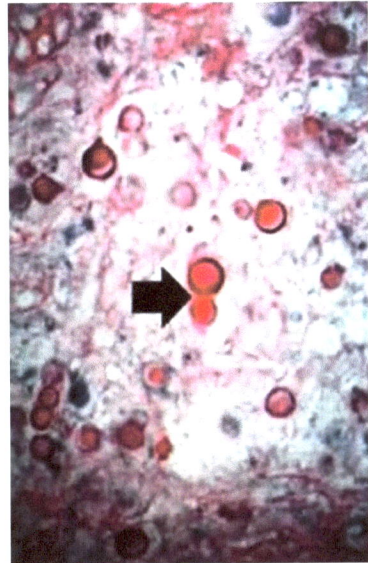

BLASTOMYCOSIS
PAS stain of tissue section showing **budding** yeast-like cells of *B. dermatitidis* [Interactive Pathology Lab.: peir. path. uab. edu/ iplab/]

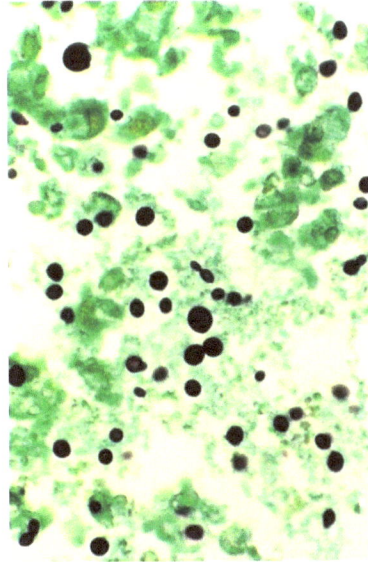

CRYPTOCOCCOSIS
Histopathology of lung section of an AIDS patient showing numerous extracellular yeasts of *Cryptococcus neoformans* within alveolar spaces (*wikipedia.org/*)

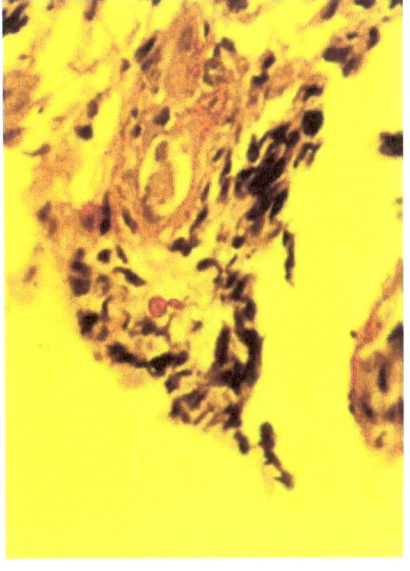

SPOROTHRICOSIS
PAS stain showing positive budding yeast-like cells of *Sporothrix schenckii* in tissue [mycology.adelaide.edu.au]

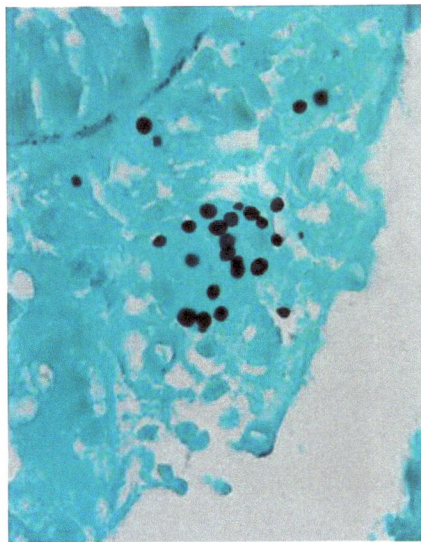

HISTOPLASMOSIS
GMS of tissue section showing yeast form of *Histoplasma capsulatum* (dark) *[mycology.adelaide.edu.au]*

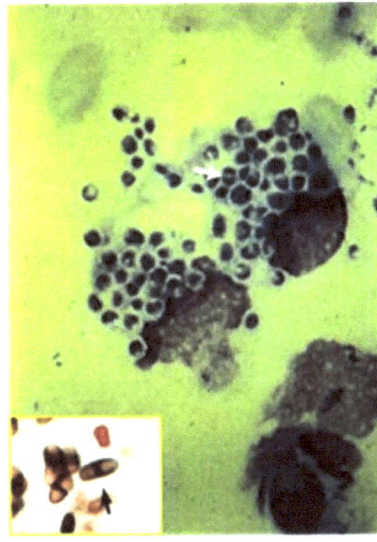

PENICILLIOSIS
Yeast-cells spherical divide by fission of *P. marneffei* in an HIV patient with generalized papular rash (*www. med. cmu. ac. th/ l*)

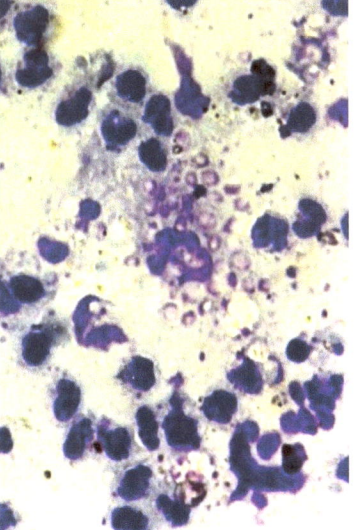

HISTOPLASMOSIS
H. capsulatum in cytoplasm of a macrophage, fine-needle aspirate from a horse lymph node (Giemsa)

PRESENCE OF HYPHAE

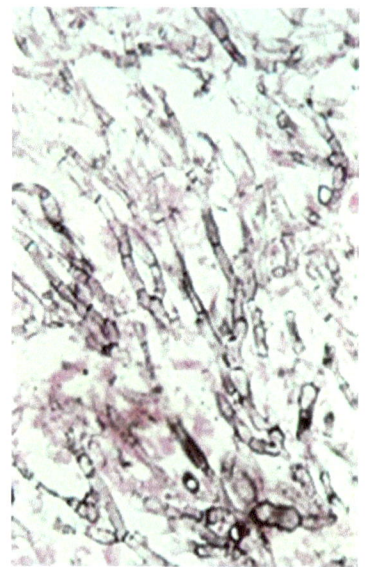

FUNGAL HYPHAE
H&E stained section of tissue showing hyaline septate hyphae suggesting fungal infection [mycology.adelaide.edu.au]

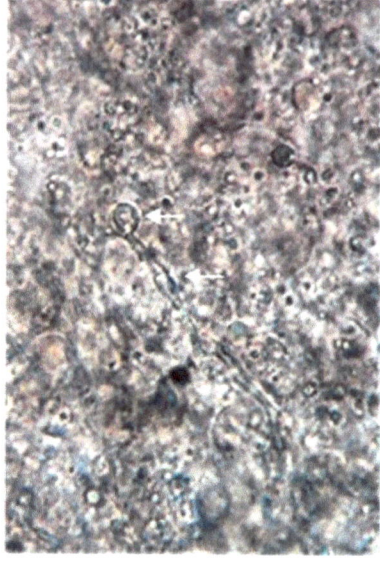

ASPERGILLOSIS
KOH mount from pus of a brain abscess showing fungal hyphae and vesicle suggesting aspergillosis

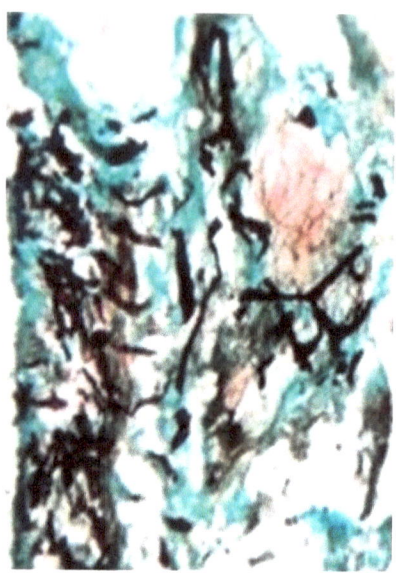

FUNGAL HYPHAE
GMS stain of bone marrow space showing fungal hyphae [www.ispub.com/journal/the_internet_journal_of_dental_science/vol. 6, No. 2, 25]

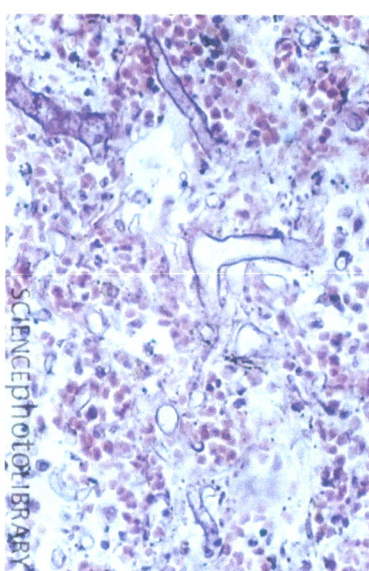

ZYGOMYCOSIS
H&E stained section of infected tissue showing broad hyphae caused by *Mucor* sp. (*CNRI/Science Photo Library*)

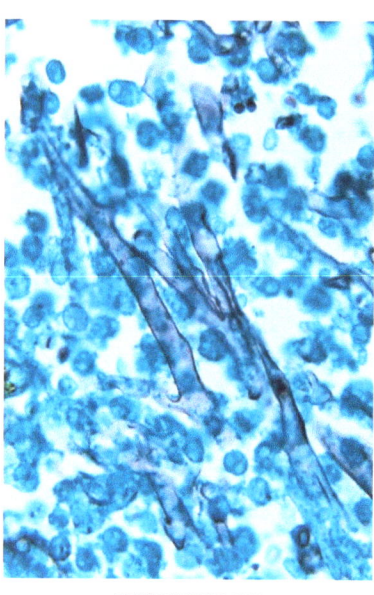

ZYGOMYCOSIS
GMS stained section of infected tissue showing broad hyphae caused by *Mucor pusilluss* [CDC/Dr. Libero Ajello] zygomycosis). Sections of non-septate fungal hyphae (tubular shapes) are seen

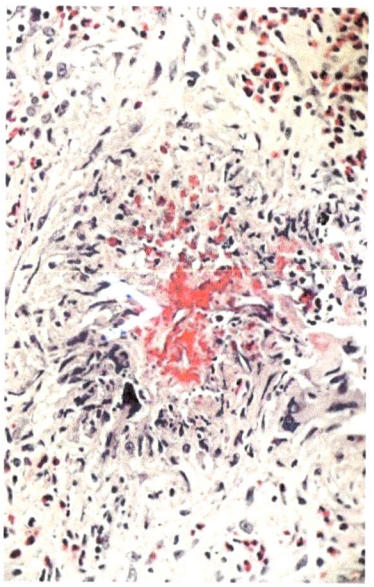

ZYGOMYCOSIS
H&E stained section of infected abdominal tissue showing broad hyphae surrounded by an eosinophilic sheath typical of zygomycosis (*Basidiobolus sp.*)

PRESENCE OF PSEUDOHYPHAE AND YEAST CELLS

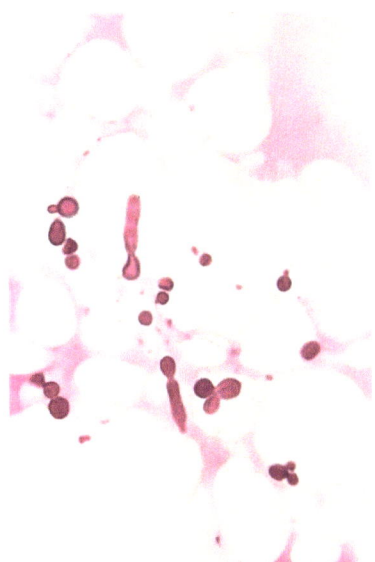

TINEA VERSICOLOR
Malassezia furfur in skin scale from a patient with tinea versicolor showing bottle neck shape budding cells and long herm tube like pseudohyphae (H &E) (*wikipedia. org/*)

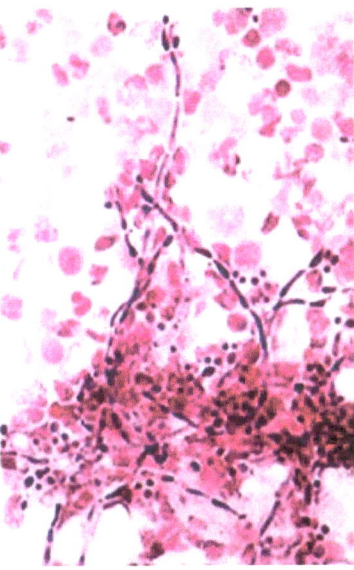

CANDIDIASIS (urine)
PAS stained smear showing the presence of budding yeast cells and pseudohyphae in a urine specimen [*www.pharmag8.com*]

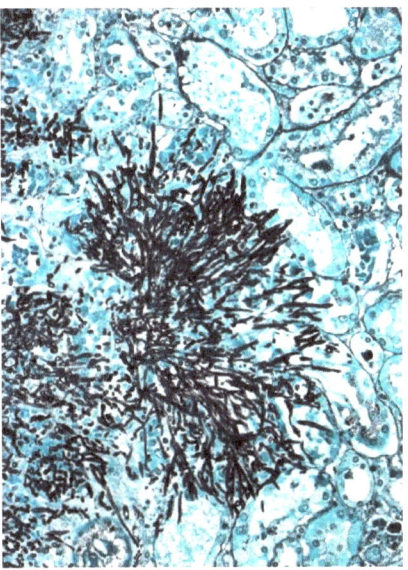

TRICHOSPORONOSIS
GMS stained section from lung with disseminated trichosporonosis showing fungal mass of budding yeasts and pseudohyphae (*humanpath.com*)

PRESENCE OF SPHERULES

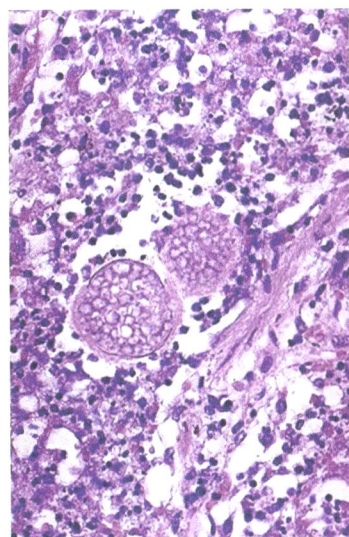

COCCIDIOIDOMYCOSIS
PAS stain of lung tissue showing **spherules** of *Coccidioides immits* [*http://infectionnet.org//*]

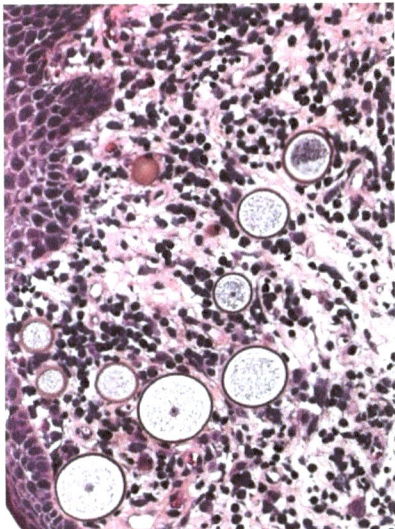

RHINOSPORIDIOSIS
Sporangia of *Rhinosporidium seeberi* within nasal polyp resembling **spherules** of *Coccidioides* (PAS) (*humpath.com*)

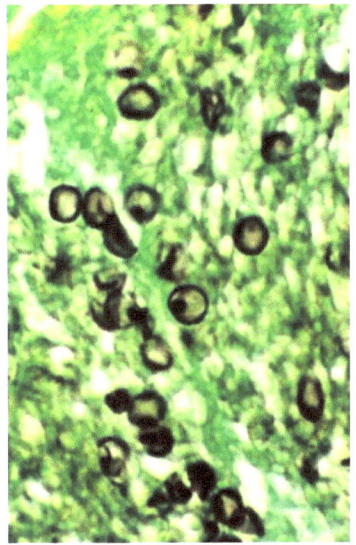

PNEUMOCYSTIS PNEUMONIA
Section of lung tissue (green) with *Pneumocystis jiroveci* **cysts** (dark spheres) stained with GMS (*CDC Public Health Image Library*)

PRESENCE OF SCLEROTIC BODIES

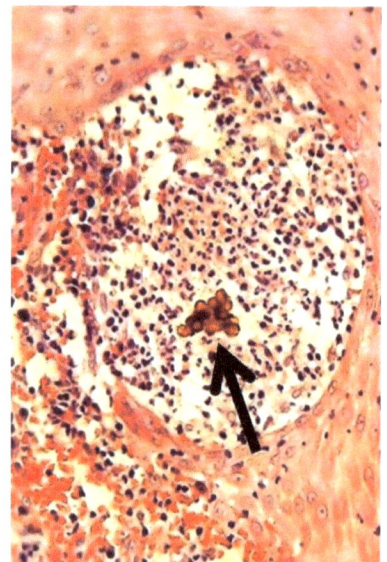

CHROMOBLASTOMYCOSIS
H&E stained tissue section showing **brown sclerotic** bodies characteristic for chromoblastomycosis (H&E)
[*Chris Alipo; www. flickr. com/ photos/ lordzagato/*]

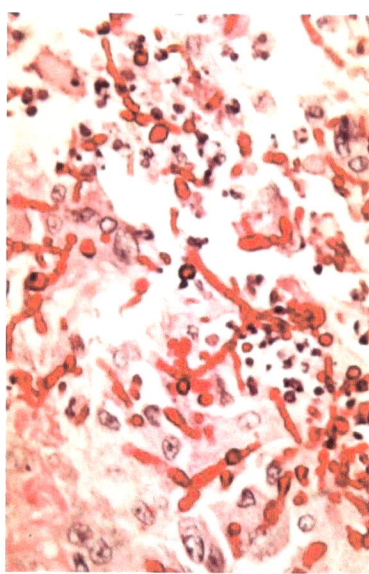

PHAEOHYPHOMYCOSIS
Phaeohyphomycosis caused by *Exophiala jeanselmei*. Note dark-walled fungi that form pigmented hyphae, or fine branching tubes, and yeast like cells in the infected tissues (*microbeworld.or*)

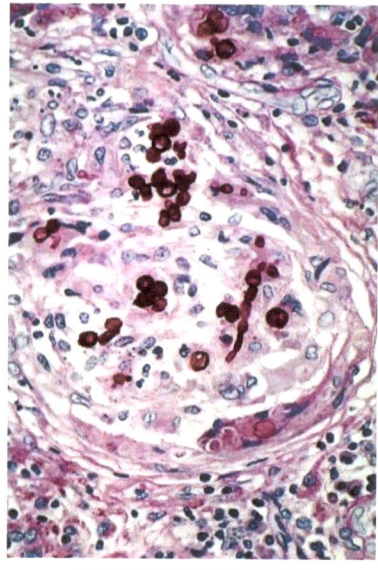

PHAEOHYPHOMYCOSIS
Phaeohyphomycosis caused by *Wangiella dermatitidis*. Note dark-walled fungi that form pigmented hyphae, or fine branching tubes, and yeast like (*ru.wikipedia.org*) cells in the infected tissues

PRESENCE OF GRAINS

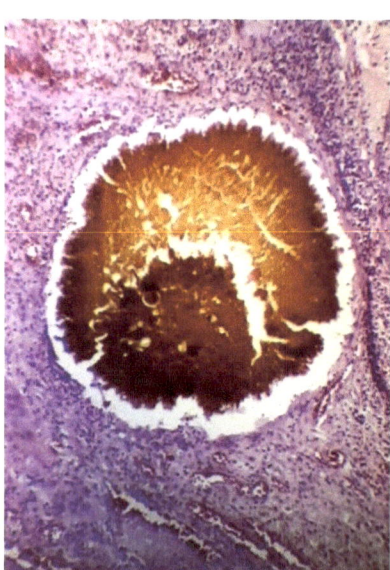

MYCETOMA (eumycotic)
Subcutaneous nodule showing black grained mycetoma caused by *Madurella mycetomatis* (H&E)
[*www.thailabonline.com/*]

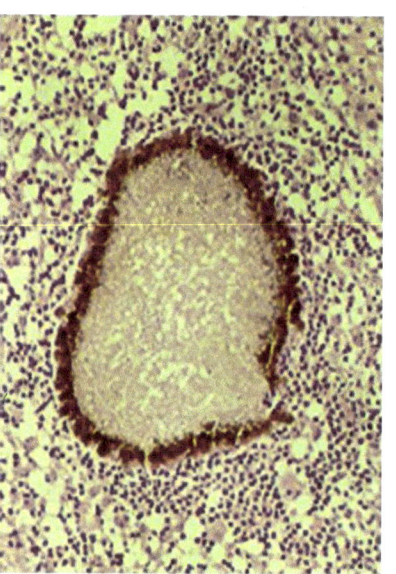

MYCETOMA (eumycotic)
H&E stained tissue section showing black grained eumycotic mycetoma caused by *Madurella mycetomatis*
[*mycology.adelaide.edu.au*]

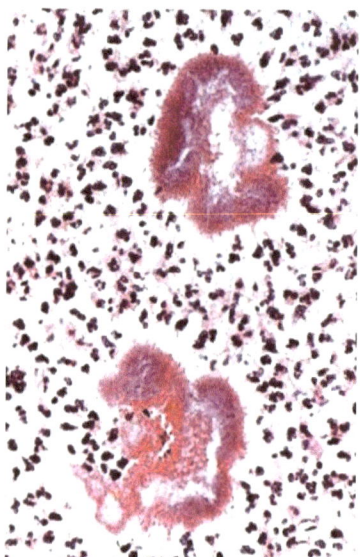

MYCETOMA (actinomycetoma)
Grains and filaments in abscess in actinomycetoma caused by *Nocardia brasiliensis* (H&E)
(*otm. oxfordmedicine. com*)

SECTION TWO: COLLECTION, PROCESSING, MICROSCOPY AND CULTURE OF CLINICAL SPECIMENS

SKIN, HAIR AND NAILS

Specimen collection: Wipe lesions with alcohol sponge or sterile water, scrape the entire lesion (s) with a sterile scalpel, and place scrapings (nails, hair or scales) in a clean Petri dish labeled with the patient's data. Transport to the laboratory, discard remaining pieces of the collection device at the patient's bedside. Send specimen to the lab. ASAP or keep at **room temperature** [*moisten with sterile normal saline to avoid dryness*]
Processing: Process the specimen by mincing it into pieces as small as possible with a sterile scalpel blade by grinding in a sterile glass tissue grinder. Inoculate the homogenized material onto the media listed below. Then perform a smear for direct microscopic examinations.

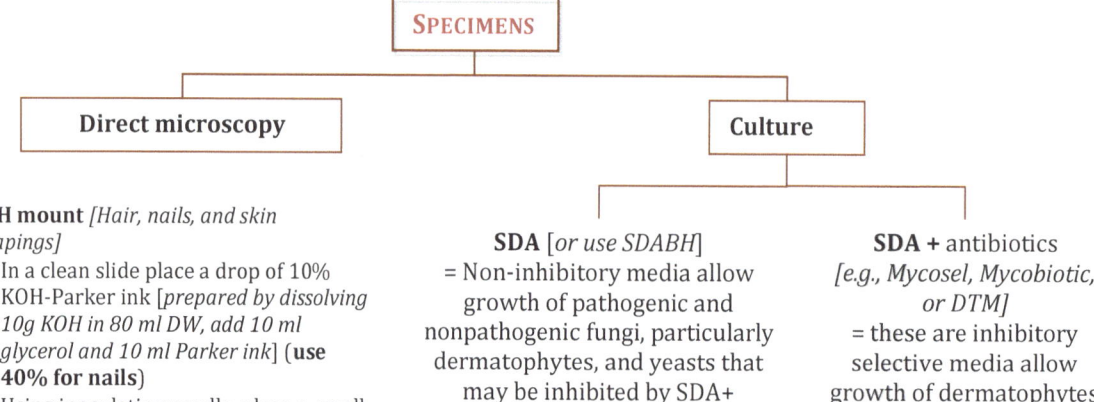

KOH mount *[Hair, nails, and skin scrapings]*
- In a clean slide place a drop of 10% KOH-Parker ink [*prepared by dissolving 10g KOH in 80 ml DW, add 10 ml glycerol and 10 ml Parker ink*] (**use 40% for nails**)
- Using inoculating needle, place a small portion of specimen in the KOH drop
- Place a cover slide and squash gently, Blot off excess fluid
- Gently heat by passing 2-4 times through flame [don't boil]to allow digestion of specimen
- Wait 20 min [several hours for nails]
- Apply fingernail at the margin of the cover slide to prevent dryness of slide
- Examine microscopically for faintly blue stained fungal elements
- Negative specimen should be kept and re-examined after 1 hour or next day
(Digestion of skin sample can be done in a small tube then one drop is transferred to the slide, 1-2 drops of LPCB or Parker ink added, mixed, cover slide place and examined)

SDA [*or use SDABH*]
= Non-inhibitory media allow growth of pathogenic and nonpathogenic fungi, particularly dermatophytes, and yeasts that may be inhibited by SDA+ antibiotics

SDA + antibiotics *[e.g., Mycosel, Mycobiotic, or DTM]*
= these are inhibitory selective media allow growth of dermatophytes

Inoculation
- Using inoculating needle, **place** a small portion (2-5 hairs or a nail or scales) onto the centre of each of the above media

Don't streak specimen!
- Incubate the plates or bottles with agar **side up** in a **humid** chamber at **30ºC** (*preferably one at 26ºC [molds] and another at 35ºC [yeasts]*)[*provide humidity by a water container in the incubator*]
- Examine the culture after **3 days** then weekly for up to **6 weeks** before reporting the negative growth

Indirect microscopy
- Prepare a mount from the grown culture for indirect microscopy using either: Cellotape, Tease mount technique, Microculture technique (*see Section Five for details*)
- Stain with LPCB or Parker ink or CW (*see Section Five for details*)

COMMONLY ISOLATED SPECIES AND DISEASES THEY CAUSE

Species	**Type**	**Disease**
Dermatophytes *(Trichophyton, Microsporum, Epidermophyton)*	Molds	Dermatophytosis (tinea, ringworm)
Malassezia furfur	Yeast	Pityriasis versicolor (tinea)
Candida albicans	Yeast	Skin candidiasis
Exophiala werneckii	Mold	Tinea nigra
Trichosporon beigelii	Yeast	White piedra

SPUTUM AND OTHER RESPIRATORY SPECIMENS

Specimen collection: Collect the first **morning, 2-10 m**L sputum, ask patient to rinse mouth then collect sputum resulting from a **deep cough**, or if necessary by induction, patient expectorate immediately into a sputum collection container. *Do not let patient hold sputum in the mouth.* Place cap on, tighten, label, and transport to the laboratory, Discard remaining pieces of the collection device at the patient's bedside. Send specimen to the lab ASAP or keep at **4°C** [*moisten with sterile normal saline to avoid dryness*]

Processing: Inoculate loopful sputum onto the media listed below. Then perform smears for direct microscopic examination

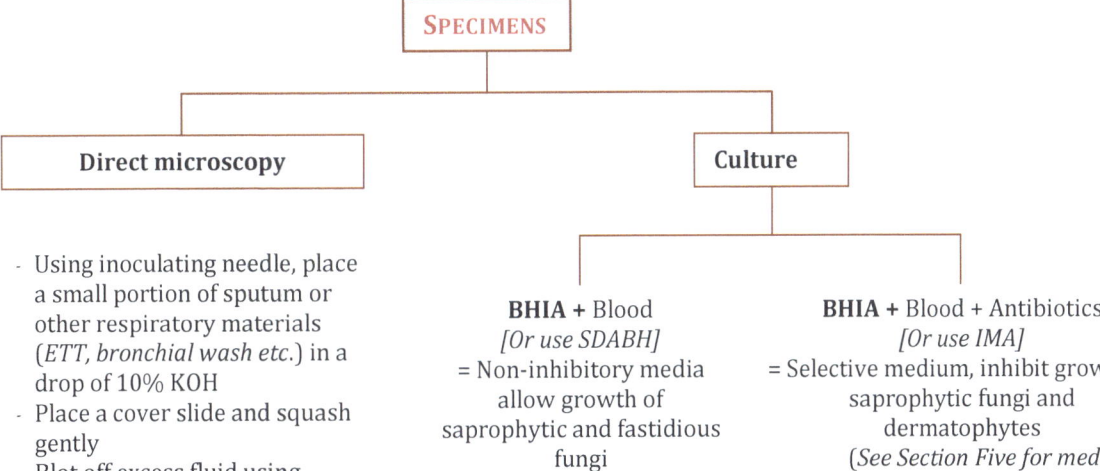

- Using inoculating needle, place a small portion of sputum or other respiratory materials (*ETT, bronchial wash etc.*) in a drop of 10% KOH
- Place a cover slide and squash gently
- Blot off excess fluid using tissue paper
- Gently heat by passing 2-4 times through flame [*don't boil*]
- Apply fingernail at the margin of the cover slide to prevent dryness of slide
- smear for prolong use
- Wait 20 min
- Examine microscopically for faintly blue stained fungal elements
- Negative specimen should be kept and re-examine next day

BHIA + Blood
[*Or use SDABH*]
= Non-inhibitory media allow growth of saprophytic and fastidious fungi

BHIA + Blood + Antibiotics
[*Or use IMA*]
= Selective medium, inhibit growth of saprophytic fungi and dermatophytes
(*See Section Five for media details*)

Inoculation
- Using inoculating needle, place a small portion (bits of sputum) onto the centre of each of the above media
  Don't streak the specimen
- Incubate the plates/ bottles **with agar side up** in a **humid** chamber at **30°C** (*preferably one at 26°C* [*molds*] *and another at 35°C* [*yeasts*])
- Examine the culture after **3 days** then weekly for up to **4-6 weeks** before reporting the negative growth

Indirect microscopy
- Prepare a mount from the grown culture for indirect microscopy using either: Cellotape, Tease mount technique, Microculture technique (*see Section Five for details*)
- Stain with LPCB or Parker ink or CW (*see Section Five for details*)

COMMONLY ISOLATED SPECIES AND DISEASES THEY CAUSE

Species	Type	Disease
Aspergillus spp.	Molds	Fungal pneumonia (Aspergillosis)
Cryptococcus neoformans	Yeast	Fungal pneumonia
Histoplasma capsulatum, Blastomyces dermatitidis, Coccidioides immitis, Paracoccidioides brasiliensis	Dimorphic fungi	Histoplasmosis and other mycosis (Fungal pneumonia)
Candida albicans	Yeast	Candidiasis
Phycomyces spp.	Molds	Phycomycosis

TISSUE BIOPSY

Specimen collection: Fresh tissue obtained at surgical biopsy is preferable to material obtained by fine needle aspiration. Sufficient specimen should be collected to allow histological examination as well as microbiological studies. Tissue is aseptically or surgically collected from the center and edge of the lesion. Place between moist gauze squares; add a small amount of sterile water or sterile normal saline to keep tissue from drying out. Send specimen to the lab ASAP or keep at **4ºC**.

Processing: Process the specimen by mincing it into pieces as small as possible with a sterile scalpel blade or by grinding in a sterile glass tissue grinder. Inoculate the homogenized material onto the same media listed below. Then perform a smear for direct microscopic examinations

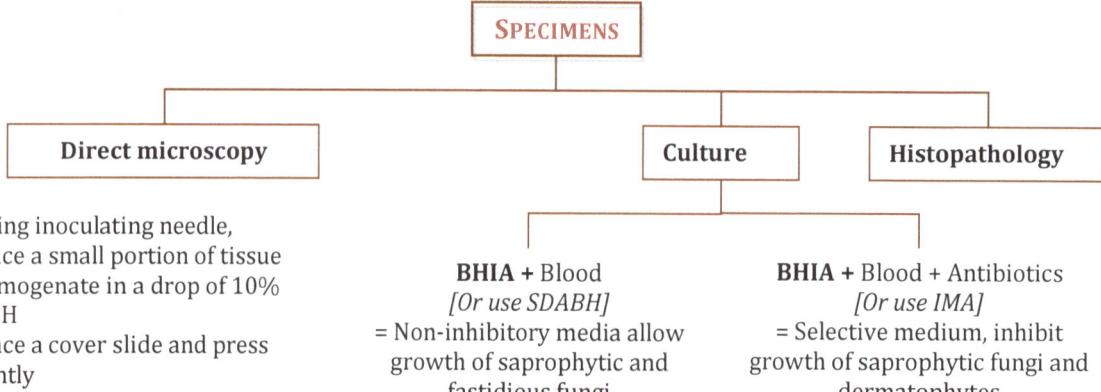

Direct microscopy
- Using inoculating needle, place a small portion of tissue homogenate in a drop of 10% KOH
- Place a cover slide and press gently
- Blot off excess fluid
- Gently heat by passing 2-4 times through flame *[don't boil]*, apply fingernail to keep smear for prolong use
- Wait 20 min
- Examine microscopically for faintly blue stained fungal elements
- Negative specimen should be kept and re-examine next day

Culture

BHIA + Blood
[Or use SDABH]
= Non-inhibitory media allow growth of saprophytic and fastidious fungi

BHIA + Blood + Antibiotics
[Or use IMA]
= Selective medium, inhibit growth of saprophytic fungi and dermatophytes

Inoculation
- Using inoculating needle, place a small portion of tissue in duplicate onto each of the above media, **DON'T STREAK**
- Incubate the plates/ bottles **with agar side up** in a **humid** chamber at **30ºC** (*preferably one at 26ºC* [molds] *and another at 35ºC* [yeasts])
- Examine the culture after **3 days** then weekly for up to **6 weeks** before reporting the negative growth

Indirect microscopy
- Prepare a mount from the grown culture for indirect microscopy using either: Cellotape, Tease mount technique or Microculture technique (*see Section Five for details*)
- Stain with LPCB or Parker ink or CW (*see Section Five for details*)

COMMONLY ISOLATED SPECIES AND DISEASES THEY CAUSE

Species	Type	Disease
Sporothrix schenkii	Dimorphic	Sporothricosis
Madurella spp.	Molds	Mycetoma
Cladosporium sp.	Mold	Chromoblastomycosis
Rhizopus spp., *Mucor* spp.	Molds	Zygomycosis
Blastomyces dermatitidis, Coccidioides immitis, Paracoccidioides brasiliensis	Dimorphic fungi	Cutaneous mycosis
Aspergillus spp.	Molds	Aspergillosis
Candida albicans	Yeast	Candidiasis

BLOOD AND BONE MARROW

Specimen collection: Clean the area with disinfectant (70% alcohol, 1-2% iodine) at the time of collection. Use 0.05% sodium polyethanol sulfonate as an anticoagulant [Adults: 20-30 mL; Children: 1-5 mL]. Send to lab. ASAP (deliver to the lab within 2 hours of collection). Store at 30-37°C if short delay in processing is anticipated.

Processing: Prepare smears for Giemsa, Gram or PAS for staining; the remaining 3-5 mL of bone marrow and blood may be cultured on the media listed below. Inoculate 0.5-1.0 ml of puffy coat, prepared by centrifuging 5-10 mL of blood, onto the surface of the media listed below

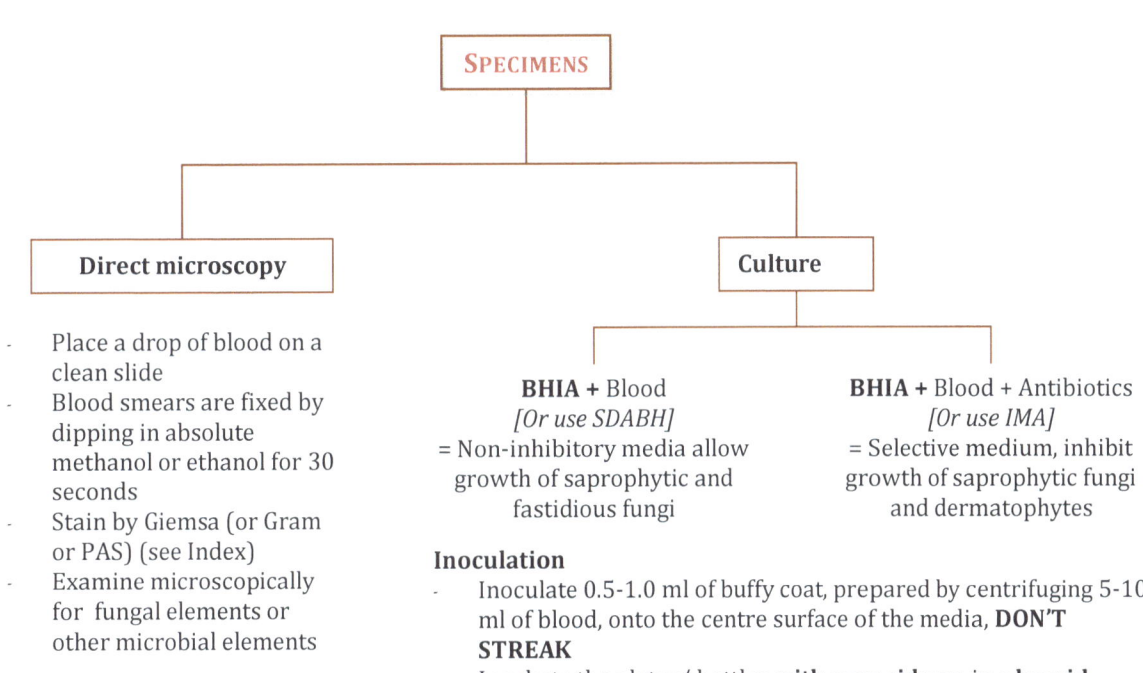

Direct microscopy

- Place a drop of blood on a clean slide
- Blood smears are fixed by dipping in absolute methanol or ethanol for 30 seconds
- Stain by Giemsa (or Gram or PAS) (see Index)
- Examine microscopically for fungal elements or other microbial elements

Culture

BHIA + Blood *[Or use SDABH]* = Non-inhibitory media allow growth of saprophytic and fastidious fungi

BHIA + Blood + Antibiotics *[Or use IMA]* = Selective medium, inhibit growth of saprophytic fungi and dermatophytes

Inoculation
- Inoculate 0.5-1.0 ml of buffy coat, prepared by centrifuging 5-10 ml of blood, onto the centre surface of the media, **DON'T STREAK**
- Incubate the plates/ bottles **with agar side up** in a **humid** chamber at **30°C** (*preferably one at 26°C* [molds] *and another at 35°C* [yeasts])
- Examine the culture after **3 days** then weekly for up to **6 weeks** before reporting the negative growth

Indirect microscopy
- Prepare a mount from the grown culture for indirect microscopy using either: Cellotape, Tease mount technique or Microculture technique (*see Section Five for details*)
- Stain with LPCB or Parker ink or CW (*see Section Five for details*)
- Stain with LPCB or Parker ink or CW (*see Section Five for details*)

COMMONLY ISOLATED SPECIES AND DISEASES THEY CAUSE

Species	Type	Disease
Candida albicans	Yeast	Endocarditis
Aspergillus spp.	Molds	Aspergillosis

CSF AND BRAIN ABSCESS ASPIRATE

Specimen collection Specimen collected by physician in a sterile screw capped or snap cap tubes. Collect 3-5 mL of CSF /aspirate. Handle as a STAT (immediately). If there is delay keep specimen at room temperature or incubated at 30°C *[Do not refrigerate]*

Processing: Centrifuge the specimen. Keep the supernatant for cryptococcal antigen testing and process the sediment as follows:
- For direct microscopy use 1 drop of the sediment to make an India ink mount and one drop to make a dry smear for Gram stain
- Re-suspend the remaining sediment in 1-2 ml of CSF and inoculate onto the media below

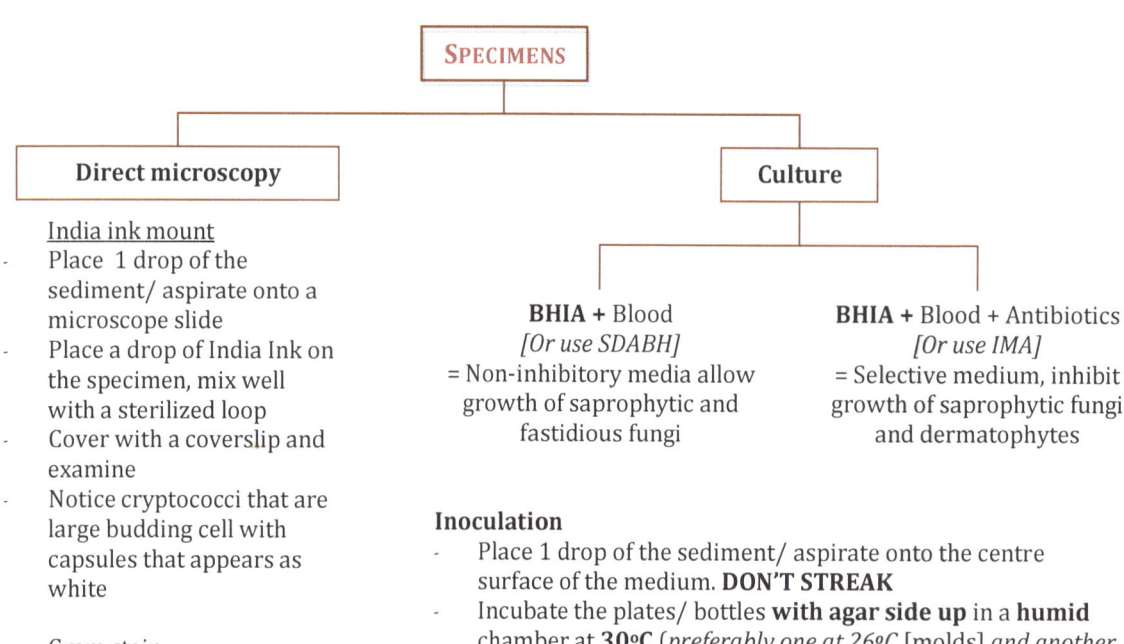

Direct microscopy

India ink mount
- Place 1 drop of the sediment/ aspirate onto a microscope slide
- Place a drop of India Ink on the specimen, mix well with a sterilized loop
- Cover with a coverslip and examine
- Notice cryptococci that are large budding cell with capsules that appears as white

Gram stain
- Stain the other slide with Gram's stain (*see Section Four*)
- Notice yeasts or Gram bacteria or inflammatory cells

Culture

BHIA + Blood
[Or use SDABH]
= Non-inhibitory media allow growth of saprophytic and fastidious fungi

BHIA + Blood + Antibiotics
[Or use IMA]
= Selective medium, inhibit growth of saprophytic fungi and dermatophytes

Inoculation
- Place 1 drop of the sediment/ aspirate onto the centre surface of the medium. **DON'T STREAK**
- Incubate the plates/ bottles **with agar side up** in a **humid** chamber at **30°C** (*preferably one at 26°C [molds] and another at 35°C [yeasts]*)
- Examine the culture after **3 days** then weekly for **4-6 weeks** before reporting the negative growth

Indirect microscopy
- Prepare a mount from the grown culture for indirect microscopy using either: Cellotape, Tease mount technique or Microculture technique (*see Section Five for details*)
- Stain with LPCB or Parker ink or CW (*see Section Five for details*)

COMMONLY ISOLATED SPECIES AND DISEASES THEY CAUSE

Species	Type	Disease
Cryptococcus neoformans	Yeast	Cryptococcosis (meningitis)
Histoplasma capsulatum, Coccidioides immitis,	Dimorphic fungi	Meningitis, cerebral abscess
Aspergillus spp.	Molds	Meningitis, cerebral abscess
Candida albicans	Yeast	Meningitis, cerebral abscess
Note: *Mycobacterium tuberculosis*	Bacteria	Chronic granulomatous meningitis

PUS, EXUDATES, GRAINS AND DRAINAGE

Specimen collection: Using a sterile needle and syringe, aspirate material [**1-5 mL**] from un-drained abscesses. Place the material in a sterile container labeled with the patient's data. Specimen may be kept moist by adding drops of sterile saline. Specimen process ASAP or keep at **4ºC** [*moisten with 0.85% sterile saline to avoid dryness*]

Processing: Process the specimen by mincing it into pieces as small as possible with a sterile scalpel blade by grinding in a sterile glass tissue grinder. Inoculate the homogenized material onto the same media listed below. Then perform a smear for direct microscopic examinations

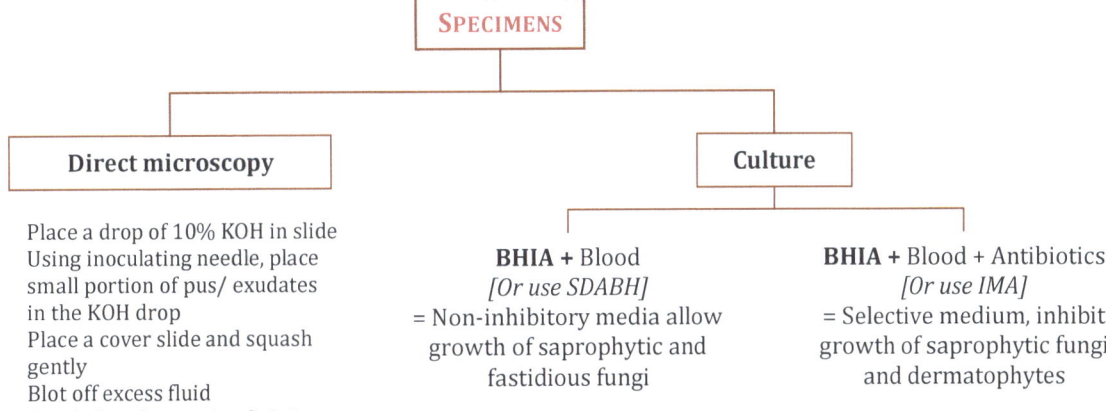

Direct microscopy
- Place a drop of 10% KOH in slide
- Using inoculating needle, place small portion of pus/ exudates in the KOH drop
- Place a cover slide and squash gently
- Blot off excess fluid
- Gently heat by passing 2-4 times through flame [*don't boil*], apply fingernail to use for prolong use
- Wait 20 min
- Examine microscopically for faintly blue stained fungal elements
- Negative specimen should be kept and re-examine next day

Culture

BHIA + Blood [*Or use SDABH*] = Non-inhibitory media allow growth of saprophytic and fastidious fungi

BHIA + Blood + Antibiotics [*Or use IMA*] = Selective medium, inhibit growth of saprophytic fungi and dermatophytes

Inoculation
- Inoculate 0.5-1.0 ml of pus/ exudates onto the surface of the medium
- Incubate plates/ bottles **with agar side up** in a **humid** chamber at **30ºC** (*preferably one at 26ºC* [molds] *and another at 35ºC* [yeasts]). **DON'T STREAK**
- Examine the culture after **3 days** then weekly for **4-6 weeks** before reporting the negative growth

Indirect microscopy
- Prepare a mount from the grown culture for indirect microscopy using either: Cellotape, Tease mount technique or Microculture technique (*see Section Five for details*)
- Stain with LPCB or Parker ink or CW (*see Section Five for details*)

COMMONLY ISOLATED SPECIES AND DISEASES THEY CAUSE

Species	**Type**	**Disease**
Cryptococcus neoformans	Yeast	Cryptococcosis
Candida albicans	Yeast	Candidiasis
Sporothrix schenkii	Dimorphic	Sporothricosis
Madurella spp.	Molds	Mycetoma
Cladosporium sp.	Mold	Chromoblastomycosis
Rhizopus spp., *Mucor* spp.	Molds	Zygomycosis
Blastomyces dermatitidis, Coccidioides immitis, Paracoccidioides brasiliensis	Dimorphic fungi	Blastomycosis, and other mycosis
Aspergillus spp.	Molds	Aspergillosis
Phialophoria sp., *Scedosporium (Pseudoallescheria)* sp.	Molds	Mycosis

VAGINAL SWAB AND DISCHARGE

Specimen collection: Using several sterile swabs, collect material from vagina (*swab or 1-5mL discharge*). Insert swabs into a sterile tube, processed ASAP (*a delay of longer than two hours at room temperature may impede the detection of some fungi*). Store at 4°C if short delay in processing is anticipated

Processing:
- Check vaginal pH (*normal =4-4.5; alkaline indicates vaginosis*)
- Prepare a <u>wet saline mount</u> of the vaginal discharge for the identification of yeast cells and mycelia and to rule out other diagnoses (*the "clue cells" of bacterial vaginosis and motile trichomonads of trichomoniasis*)
- Also, prepare a 10% KOH preparation of the vaginal discharge. This has a higher sensitivity for the identification of yeasts.
[*A gram-stained preparation may also be used. Yeasts are gram-positive*]

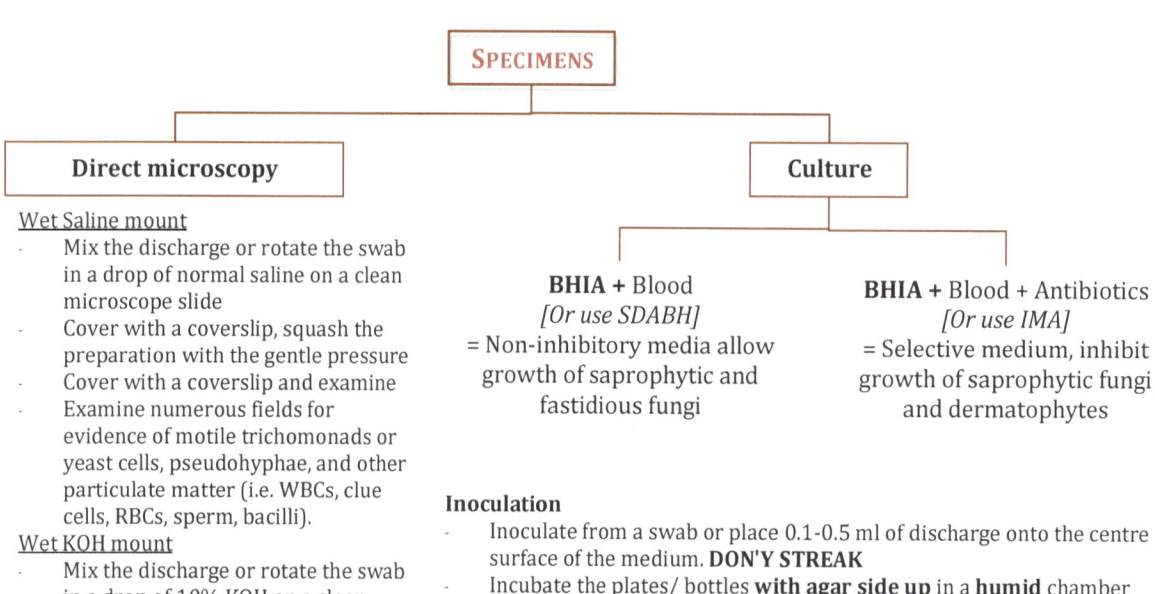

Direct microscopy

<u>Wet Saline mount</u>
- Mix the discharge or rotate the swab in a drop of normal saline on a clean microscope slide
- Cover with a coverslip, squash the preparation with the gentle pressure
- Cover with a coverslip and examine
- Examine numerous fields for evidence of motile trichomonads or yeast cells, pseudohyphae, and other particulate matter (i.e. WBCs, clue cells, RBCs, sperm, bacilli).

<u>Wet KOH mount</u>
- Mix the discharge or rotate the swab in a drop of 10% KOH on a clean microscope slide. Continue as wet saline mount above.

<u>Dry smears</u>
- Swab/ or a drop of the discharge onto a microscope slide
- Fix and let dry then stain with Gram's and examine for above mentioned organisms and cells

Culture

BHIA + Blood
[Or use SDABH]
= Non-inhibitory media allow growth of saprophytic and fastidious fungi

BHIA + Blood + Antibiotics
[Or use IMA]
= Selective medium, inhibit growth of saprophytic fungi and dermatophytes

Inoculation
- Inoculate from a swab or place 0.1-0.5 ml of discharge onto the centre surface of the medium. **DON'Y STREAK**
- Incubate the plates/ bottles **with agar side up** in a **humid** chamber at **30°C** (*preferably one at 26°C [molds] and another at 35°C [yeasts]*)
- Examine the culture after **3 days** then weekly for **4-6 weeks** before reporting the negative growth

Indirect microscopy
- Prepare a mount from the grown culture for indirect microscopy using either: Cellotape, Tease mount technique or Microculture technique (*see Section Five for details*)
- Stain with LPCB or Parker ink or CW (*see Section Five for details*)

COMMONLY ISOLATED SPECIES AND DISEASES THEY CAUSE

Species	**Type**	**Disease**
Candida albicans, Candida spp.	Yeasts	Vaginal thrush, vulvovaginal candidiasis and balanitis
Histoplasma capsulatum, Coccidioides immitis	Dimorphic fungi	Vulvovaginitis and balanitis

URINE

Specimen collection: ≥20 mL of a morning midstream clean catch urine or catheterized specimen. Processed ASAP (*a delay of longer than two hours at room temperature may impede the detection of some fungi*). Store at 4°C if short delay in processing is anticipated (*24h urine samples are unacceptable*)

Processing: Centrifuge the urine for 10-15 minutes at 2000 rpm. Decant the supernatant. Prepare a direct smear of the sediment in KOH for direct microscopy. Note PAS, Gram or India ink preparations may also be helpful. Inoculate 0.05-0.1 ml of the sediment onto the media listed below

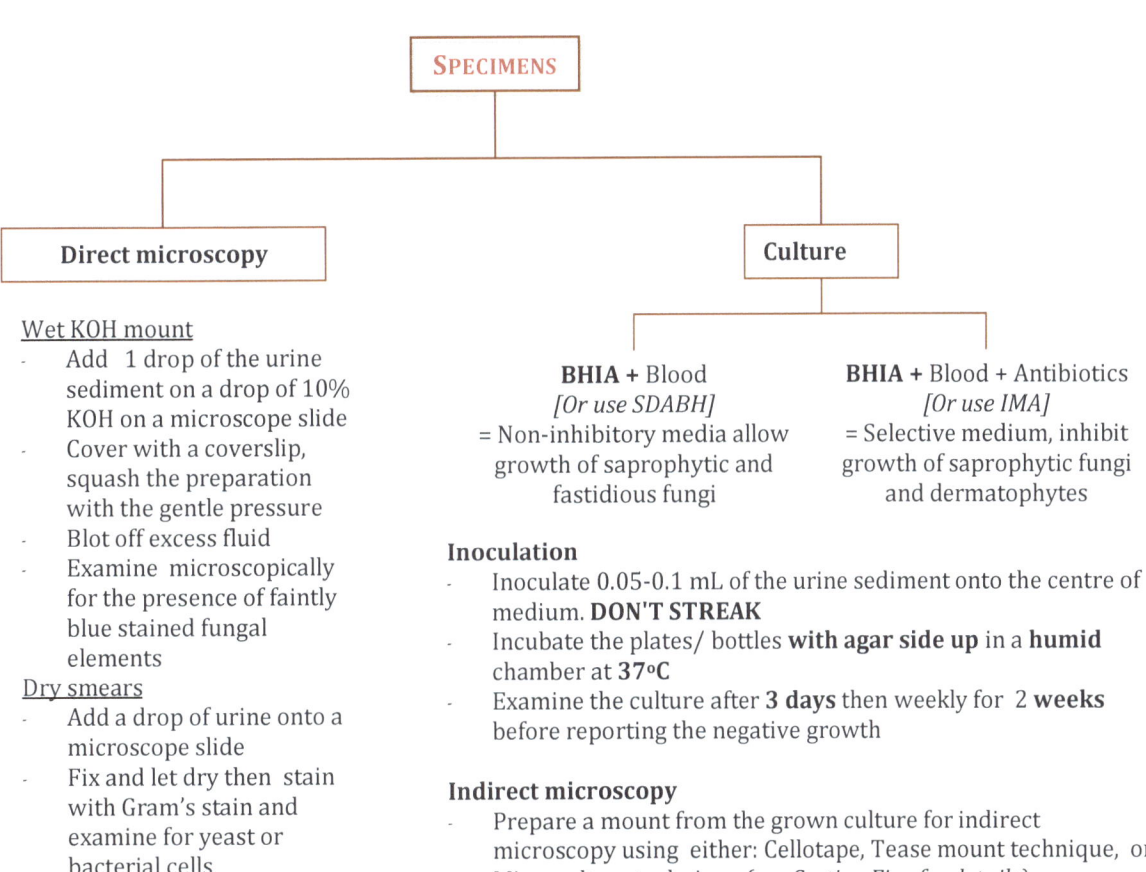

```
                          SPECIMENS
                              |
              ┌───────────────┴───────────────┐
        Direct microscopy                  Culture
```

Wet KOH mount
- Add 1 drop of the urine sediment on a drop of 10% KOH on a microscope slide
- Cover with a coverslip, squash the preparation with the gentle pressure
- Blot off excess fluid
- Examine microscopically for the presence of faintly blue stained fungal elements

Dry smears
- Add a drop of urine onto a microscope slide
- Fix and let dry then stain with Gram's stain and examine for yeast or bacterial cells

BHIA + Blood
[Or use SDABH]
= Non-inhibitory media allow growth of saprophytic and fastidious fungi

BHIA + Blood + Antibiotics
[Or use IMA]
= Selective medium, inhibit growth of saprophytic fungi and dermatophytes

Inoculation
- Inoculate 0.05-0.1 mL of the urine sediment onto the centre of medium. **DON'T STREAK**
- Incubate the plates/ bottles **with agar side up** in a **humid** chamber at **37°C**
- Examine the culture after **3 days** then weekly for **2 weeks** before reporting the negative growth

Indirect microscopy
- Prepare a mount from the grown culture for indirect microscopy using either: Cellotape, Tease mount technique, or Microculture technique (*see Section Five for details*)
- Stain with LPCB or Parker ink or CW (*see Section Five for details*)

COMMONLY ISOLATED SPECIES AND DISEASES THEY CAUSE

Species	**Type**	**Disease**
Candida albicans, Candida spp.	Yeasts	cystitis, pyelonephritis
Cryptococcus neoformans	Yeast	cystitis, pyelonephritis

SECTION THREE: SCHEMES FOR FUNGAL IDENTIFICATION

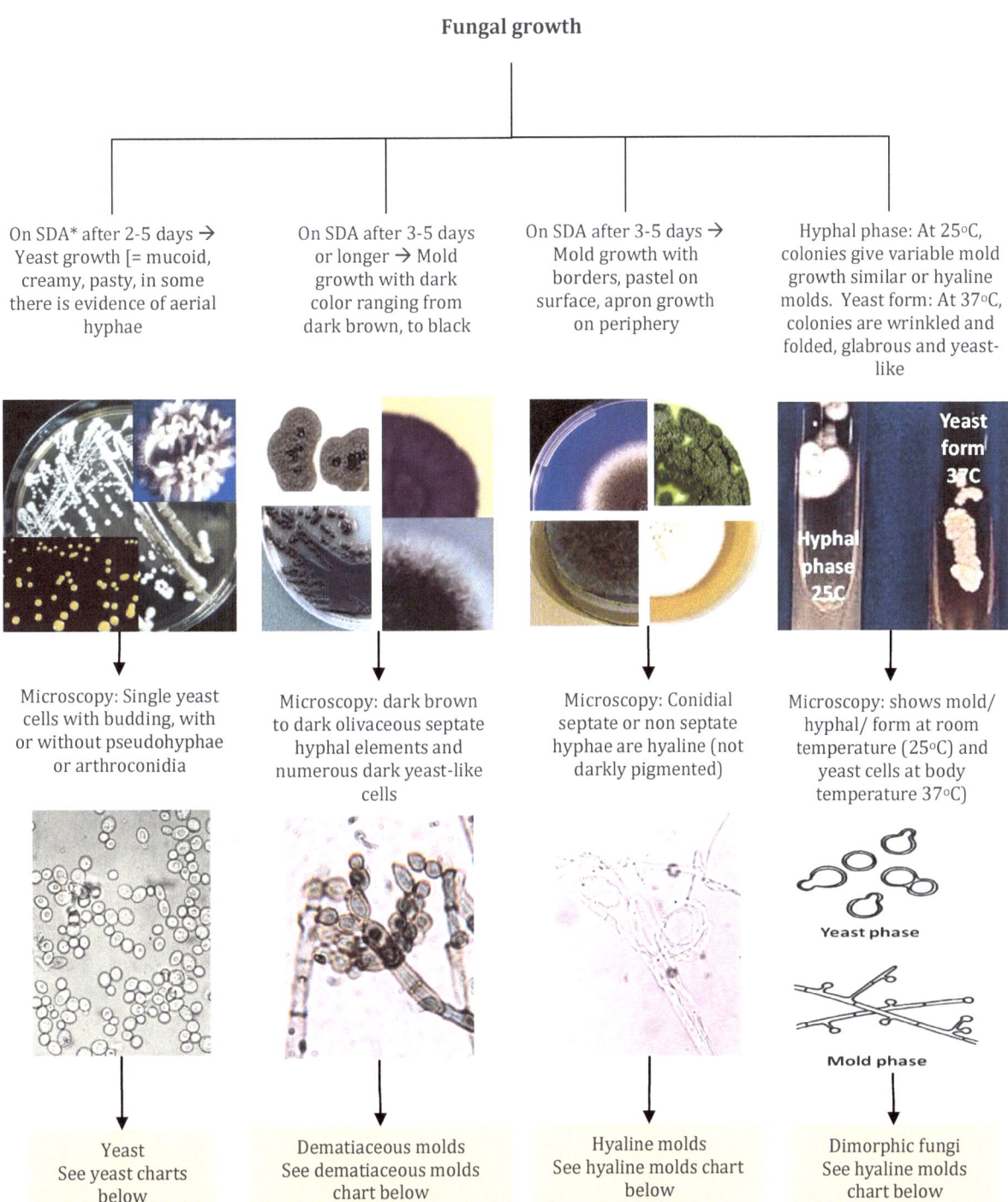

Fungal growth

- **YEASTS**
- **DEMATIACEOUS MOLDS**
- **HYALINE MOLDS**
- **DIMORPHIC FUNGI**

On SDA after 2-5 days → Yeast growth [= mucoid, creamy, pasty, in some there is evidence of aerial hyphae

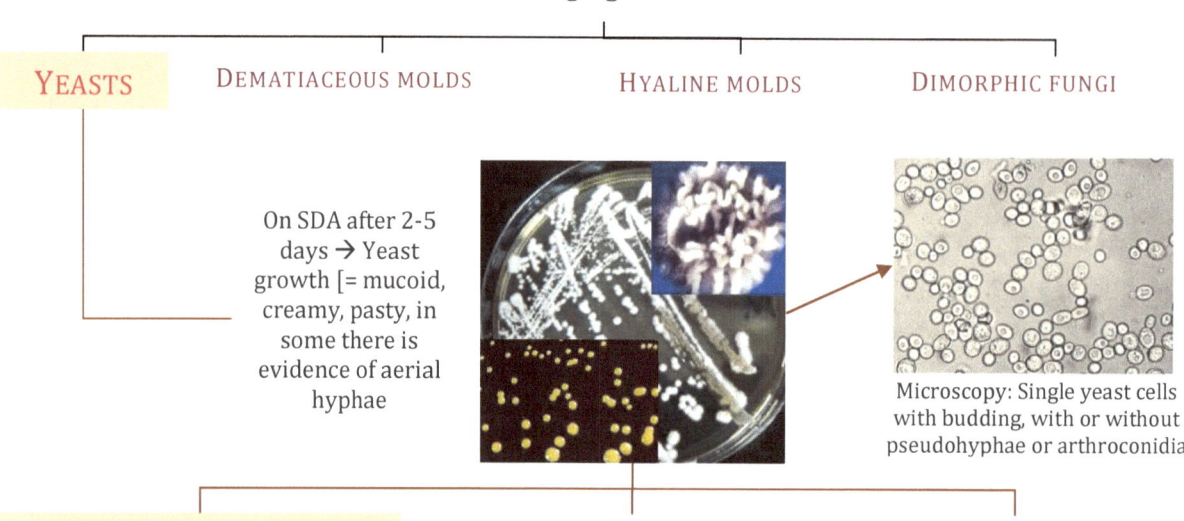

Microscopy: Single yeast cells with budding, with or without pseudohyphae or arthroconidia

Yeast cells No hyphae: *Cryptococcus, Rhodotorula, Candida glabrata, Saccharomyces*

Pseudohyphae: *Candida* spp., *Malassezia*

Hyphae and arthroconidia +/- blastoconidia: *Geotrichum, Trichosporon, Blastoschizomyces*

Rhodotorula
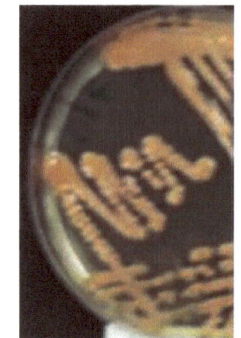
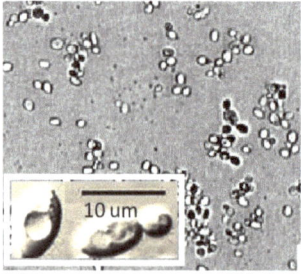

Rhodotorula
Rhodotorula is a pigmented yeast, when grown on SDA Colony color can vary from being cream colored to orange/red/pink. Microscopy: shows spherical to elongate budding yeast-like cells or blastoconidia

Cryptococcus
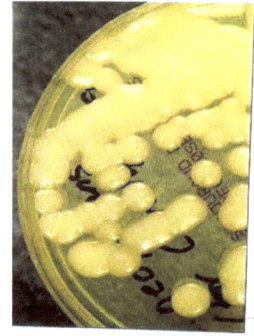
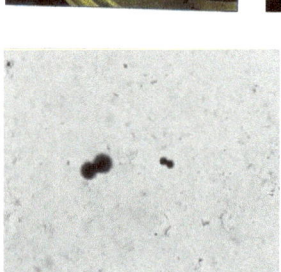

Cryptococcus neoformans
colonies are generally mucoid or slimy in appearance. Red, orange or yellow carotenoid pigments may be produced, but young colonies of most species are usually non-pigmented, and are cream in color. Microscopy: globose to elongate yeast-like cells or blastoconidia that reproduce by multilateral budding. Pseudohyphae are absent or rudimentary

Candida glabrata
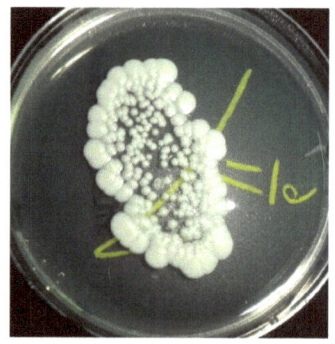
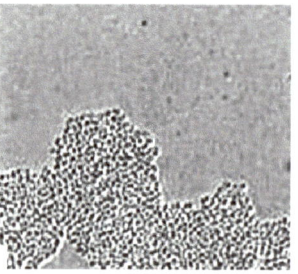

Candida glabrata
(torulopsis): Colonies are white to cream colored, smooth and glabrous yeast-like in appearance. Microscopy: shows numerous ovoid, budding yeast-like cells or blastoconidia, 2.0-4.0 x 3.0-5.5 um in size. No pseudohyphae produced

Saccharomyces
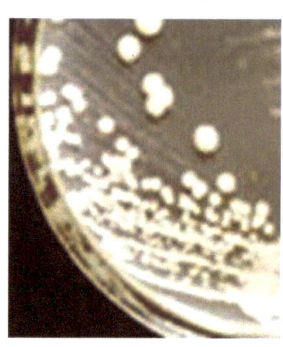
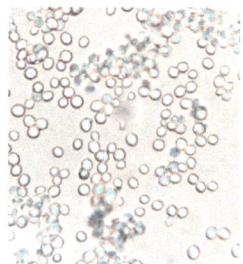

Saccharomyces cerevisiae
Colonies are white to cream colored, smooth, glabrous and yeast-like in appearance. Microscopy: shows large, globose to ellipsoidal budding yeast-like cells or blastoconidia, 3.0-10.0 x 4.5-21.0 um in size.

Fungal growth

- **YEASTS**
- DEMATIACEOUS MOLDS
- HYALINE MOLDS
- DIMORPHIC FUNGI

Yeast cell no hyphae: *Cryptococcus, Rhodotorula, C. glabrata, Saccharomyces*

Pseudohyphae: *Candida* spp., *Malassezia,*

Hyphae and arthroconidia +/- blastoconidia: *Geotrichum, Trichosporon, Blastoschizomyces*

Blastospores along long pseudohyphae *Candida* spp.

Budding yeasts & spaghetti shape hyphae and bottle shape conidia: *Malassezia* sp.

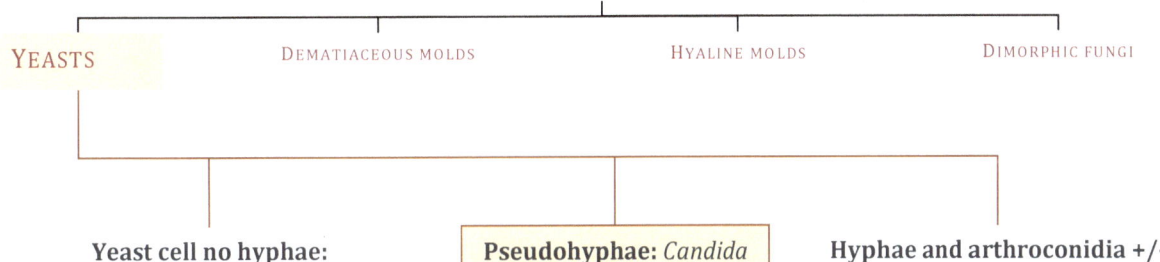

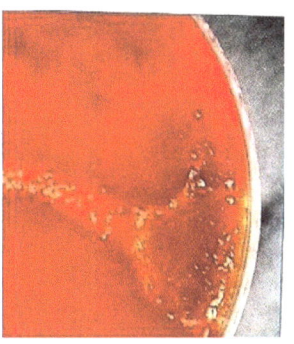

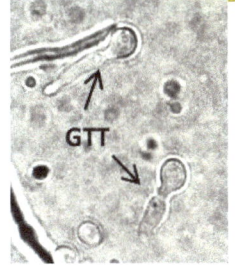
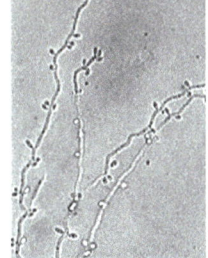
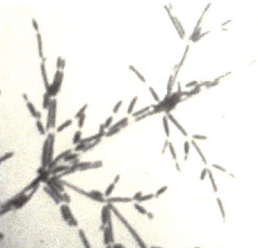

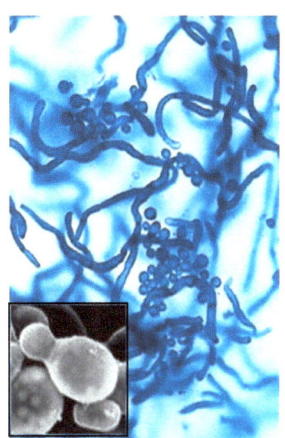

Candida albicans: colonies are white to cream colored, smooth, glabrous and yeast-like in appearance. Microscopy: shows spherical to subspherical budding yeast-like cells or blastoconidia, When incubated in serum/plasma it produces germ tube (see above)

Candida tropicalis: agar colonies are white to cream colored, smooth, glabrous and yeast-like in appearance. Microscopy: shows spherical to subspherical budding yeast-like cells or blastoconidia

Candida krusei: colonies are white to cream colored, smooth, glabrous yeast-like colonies. Microscopy: shows predominantly small, elongated to ovoid budding yeast-like cells or blastoconidia

Malassezia furfur is a lipophilic yeast (needs fatty substances). Colonies are cream to yellowish, smooth or lightly wrinkled, glistening or dull, with the margin being either entire or lobate (35-37C). Microscopy: globose, oblong-ellipsoidal to cylindrical yeast cells reproduced by budding on a broad base and from the same site at one pole (unipolar).

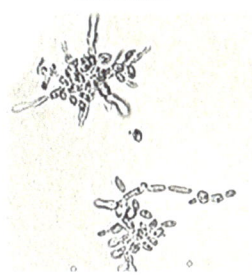
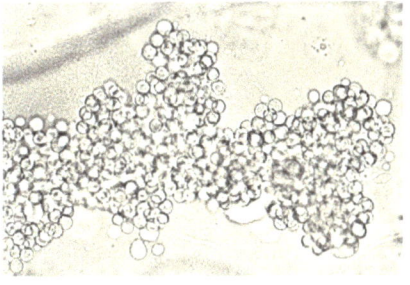

Candida parapsilosis: Colonies are white to cream colored, smooth, glabrous and yeast-like in appearance. Microscopy: shows predominantly small, globose to ovoid budding yeast-like cells or blastoconidia, 2.0-3.5 x 3.0-4.5 um in size, with some larger elongated forms present

Candida dubliniensis: Colonies are white to cream coloured, smooth, glabrous yeast-like in appearance [and are indistinguishable from those of C. albicans]. Microscopy: shows numerous ovoid, budding yeast-like cells or blastoconidia

Fungal growth

- **YEASTS**
- **DEMATIACEOUS MOLDS**
- **HYALINE MOLDS**
- **DIMORPHIC FUNGI**

Yeast cell no hyphae: Cryptococcus, Rhodotorula, C. glaborata, Saccharomyces

Pseudohyphae: Candida spp., Malassezia,

Hyphae and arthroconidia +/- blastoconidia: Geotrichum, Trichosporon, Blastoschizomyces

Blastoconidia

+ → Urease
− → *Geotrichum penicillatum* Urease negative

Urease:
- + *Trichosporon* spp.
- + *Blastoschizomyces*
- − *Geotrichum*

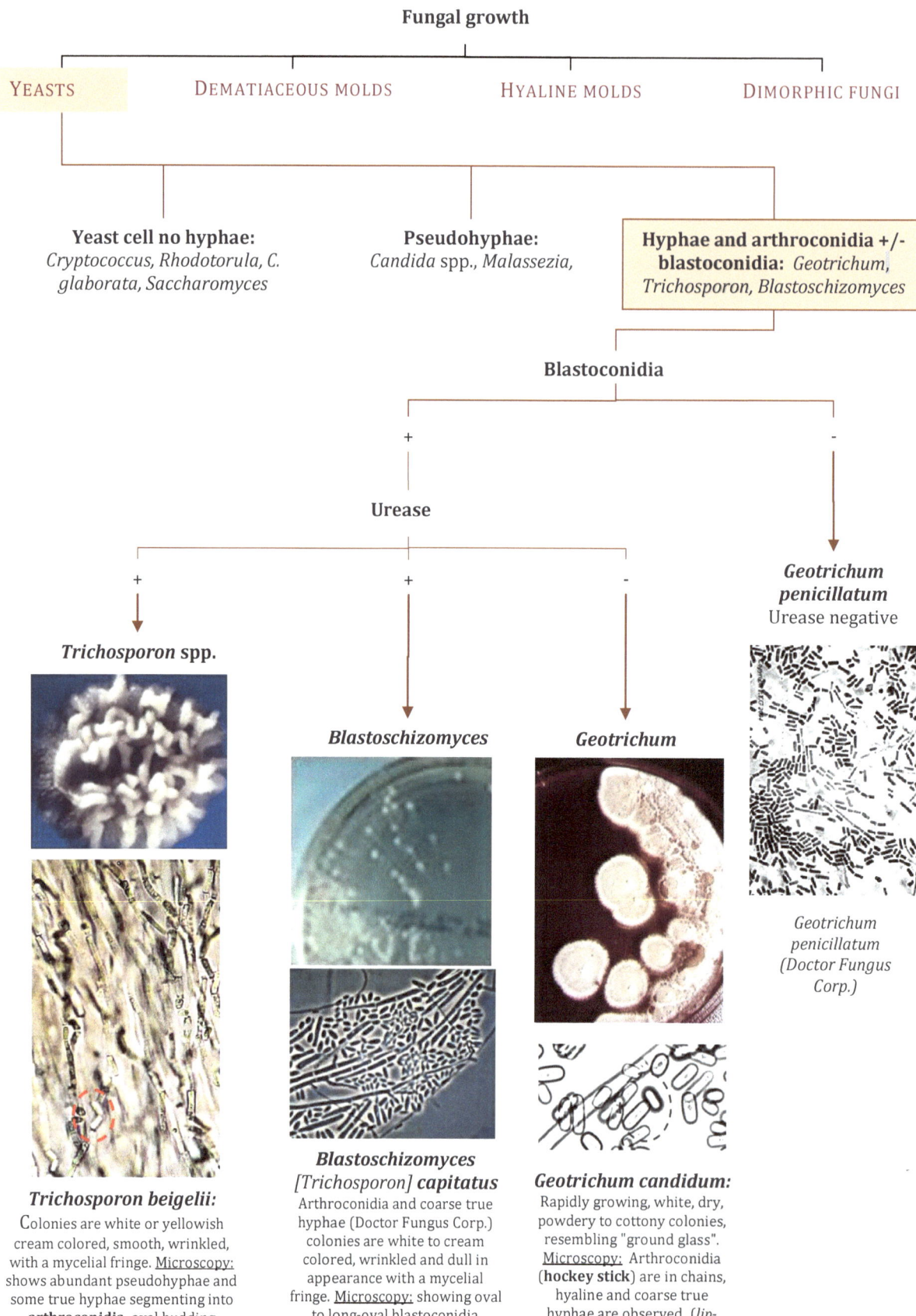

Trichosporon beigelii: Colonies are white or yellowish cream colored, smooth, wrinkled, with a mycelial fringe. Microscopy: shows abundant pseudohyphae and some true hyphae segmenting into **arthroconidia**, oval budding blastoconidia (**rabbit ear**)

Blastoschizomyces [Trichosporon] capitatus Arthroconidia and coarse true hyphae (Doctor Fungus Corp.) colonies are white to cream colored, wrinkled and dull in appearance with a mycelial fringe. Microscopy: showing oval to long-oval blastoconidia

Geotrichum candidum: Rapidly growing, white, dry, powdery to cottony colonies, resembling "ground glass". Microscopy: Arthroconidia (**hockey stick**) are in chains, hyaline and coarse true hyphae are observed. (lip-sas.fr)

Geotrichum penicillatum (Doctor Fungus Corp.)

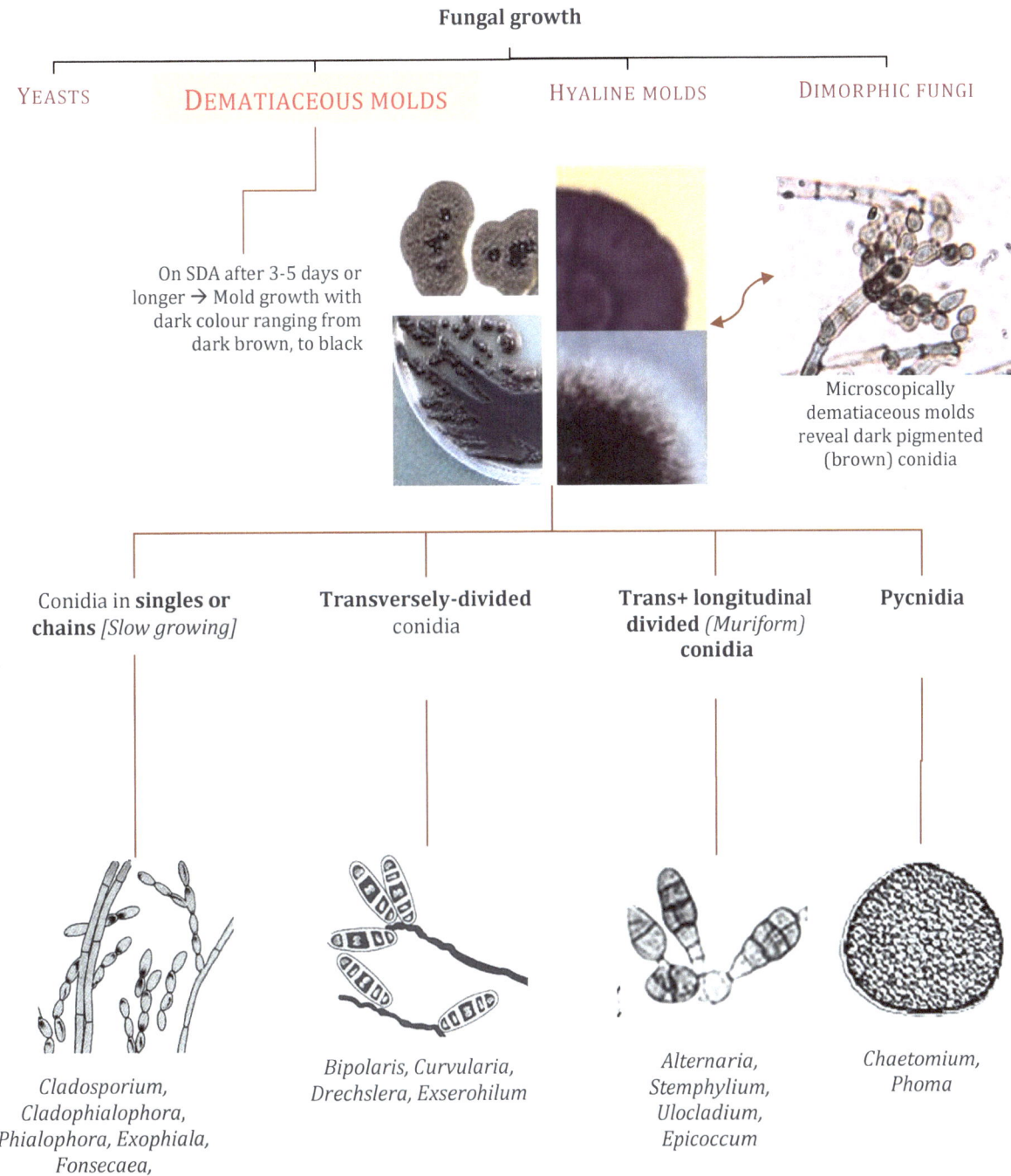

Fungal growth

- **YEASTS**
- **DEMATIACEOUS MOLDS**
- **HYALINE MOLDS**
- **DIMORPHIC FUNGI**

Dematiaceous molds

- **Conidia in singles or chains** *[Slow growing]*
  Cladosporium, Cladophialophora, Phialophora, Exophiala, Fonsecaea, Phaeoacremonium, Sporothrix, Aureobasidium, Ramichoridium, Rhinociadiella

- **Transversely-divided conidia** *Bipolaris, Curvularia, Drechslera, Exserohilum*

- **Trans+ longitudinal divided (Muriform) conidia** *Alternaria, Stemphylium, Ulocladium,* and *Epicoccum*

- **Pycnidia** *Chaetomium, Phoma*

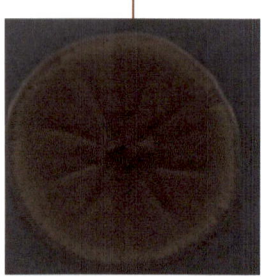
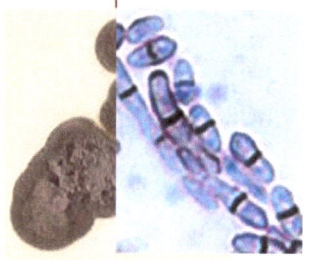
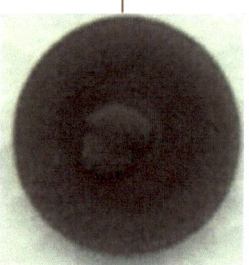
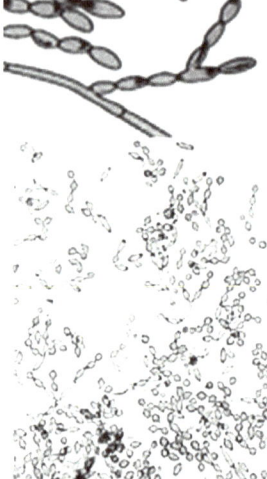
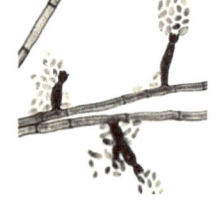
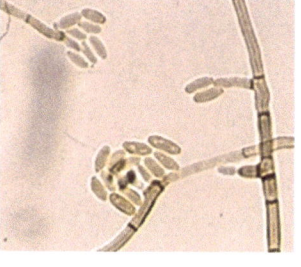
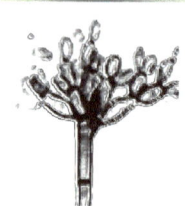

Cladophialophora, Cladosporium
Colonies is moderate at 25°C and the texture is velvety to powdery. Similar to the other dematiaceous fungi, the color is olivaceous green to black from the front and black from the reverse. Microscopy: septate brown hyphae, erect and pigmented conidiophores, and conidia

Phialophora:
Colonies grow slowly (7 days at 25°C). The texture is wooly to velvety and may be heaped and granular in some strains. From the front, the color is initially white and later becomes dark grey-green. Microscopy: Septate hyphae, phialides, and conidia are observed, hyphae are branched, and hyaline to brown

Exophiala werneckii
[*Hortaea werneckii*; *Cladosporium werneckii*] are initially yeast-like, moist, and brownish to greenish black in color. The texture of the colony eventually becomes velvety the front color is olivaceous-black and the reverse is black in mature colonies. Microscopy: yeast-like cells are visualized in long chains then septate hyphae which bear conidiogenous cells (annelides) are eventually for med. The annelides are tubular and rocket-shaped and typically taper to form a narrow elongated tip

Fonsecaea
Grows slowly and produces restricted, flat to raised and folded, velvety to cottony colonies at 25°C, when mature they are olivaceous to brown-black in color. Microscopy: septate, dark brown hyphae and suberect conidiophores that highly branch at apices. The conidiophores are pale brown, erect, septate, and sympodial with conidiogenous zones confined to the upper portion. The conidia are brown and barrel-shaped

Fungal growth

- **YEASTS**
- **DEMATIACEOUS MOLDS**
- **HYALINE MOLDS**
- **DIMORPHIC FUNGI**

Dematiaceous molds

- **Conidia in singles or chains** [Slow growing]
  Cladosporium, Cladophialophora, Phialophora, Exophiala, Fonsecaea Phaeoacremonium, Sporothrix, Aureobasidium, Ramichoridium Rhinociadiella
- **Transversely-divided** conidia *Bipolaris, Curvularia, Drechslera, Exserohilum*
- **Trans+ longitudinal divided (Muriform) conidia** *Alternaria, Stemphylium, Ulocladium, Epicoccum*
- **Pycnidia** *Chaetomium, Phoma*

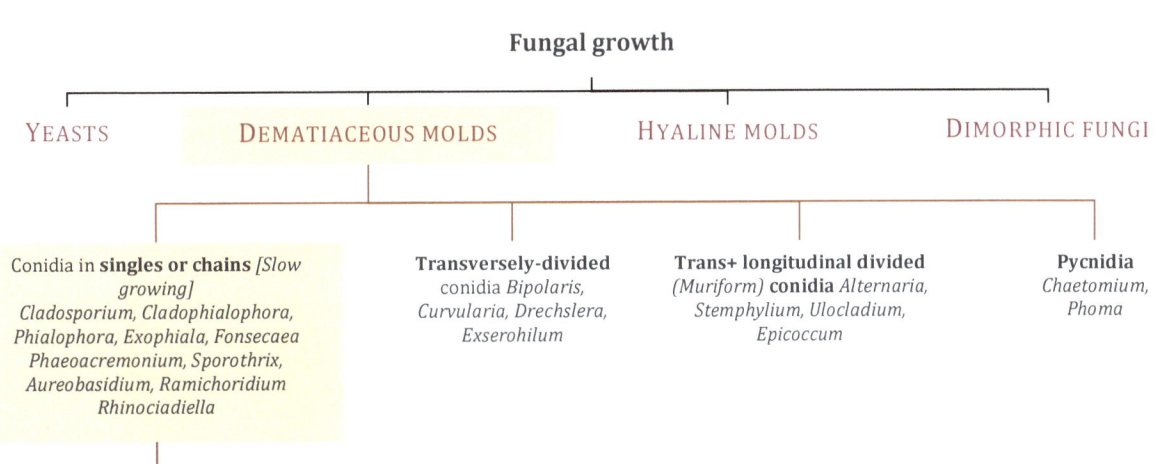
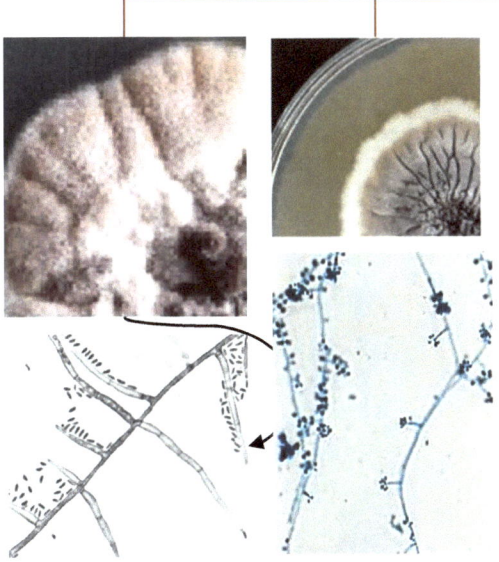
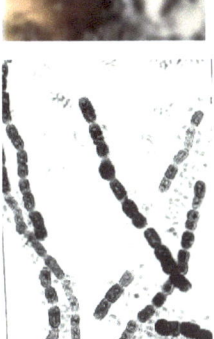
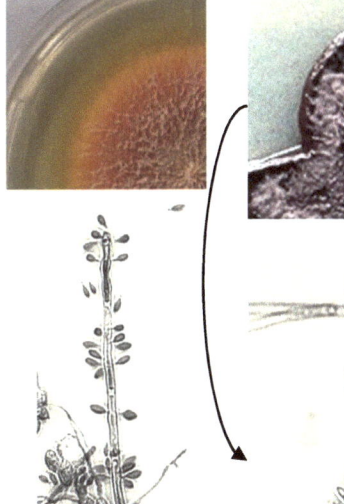
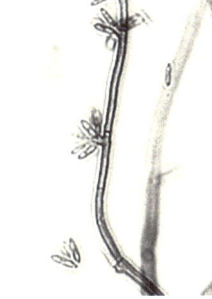

Phaeoacremonium
P. parasiticum: Cultures are slow growing, suede-like with radial furrows, initially whitish-grey becoming olivaceous-grey with age. <u>Microscopy</u>: Hyphae hyaline, later becoming brown and some becoming rough-walled. Phialides are brown, thick-walled, slender, acular to cylindrical slightly tapering towards the tip, funnel-shaped collarettes. Conidia, often in balls, are hyaline, thin-walled, cylindrical to sausage-shaped later inflating

Sporothrix (mold form)
S. schenkii: At 25C, colonies are slow growing, moist and glabrous, with a wrinkled and folded surface. Some strains may produce short aerial hyphae and pigmentation may vary from white to cream to black. On BHI blood agar at 37C, colonies are glabrous, white to greyish yellow and yeast-like, consisting of spherical or oval budding yeast cells.
<u>Microscopy</u>: Conidiophores arise at right angles from the thin septate hyphae and are usually solitary, erect and tapered towards the apex. Conidia are formed in clusters on tiny denticles by sympodial proliferation of the conidiophores [rosette-like]

Aureobasidium
A. pullulans colonies are fast growing, smooth, covered with slimy masses of conidia, cream or pink to brown or black. <u>Microscopy</u>: Hyphae are hyaline and septate frequently becoming dark-brown with age, form chains **darkly pigmented arthroconidia**.

Ramichoridium
R. schulzeri: Colonies growing rapidly, consisting of compact, flat, pale orange, brownish aerial mycelium; reverse pink to orange. <u>Microscopy</u>: Conidiophores are erect, straight, un-branched, thick-walled, reddish-brown, gradually becoming paler towards the apex, elongating sympodially with scattered, pimple-shaped conidium bearing denticles which have unpigmented scars

Rhinocladiella
R. atrovirens: Colonies are restricted, velvety or lanose, olivaceous, slightly mucoid at the centre; reverse dark olivaceous.
<u>Microscopy</u>: Conidiophores are short, brown, thick-walled. denticulate are long, with crowded, flat or butt-shaped, un pigmented conidial denticles. Conidia are hyaline, thin- smooth-walled, cylindrical, with truncate basal scars

Fungal growth

- YEASTS
- **DEMATIACEOUS MOLDS**
- HYALINE MOLDS
- DIMORPHIC FUNGI

Under **Dematiaceous molds**:

- Conidia in **singles or chains** *[Slow growing]* — *Cladosporium, Cladophialophora, Phialophora, Exophiala, Fonsecaea Phaeoacremonium, Sporothrix, Aureobasidium, Ramichoridium Rhinocladiella*
- **Transversely-divided** conidia *Bipolaris, Curvularia, Drechslera, Exserohilum*
- **Trans+ longitudinal divided** *(Muriform)* **conidia** *Alternaria, Stemphylium, Ulocladium, Epicoccum*
- **Pycnidia** *Chaetomium, Phoma*

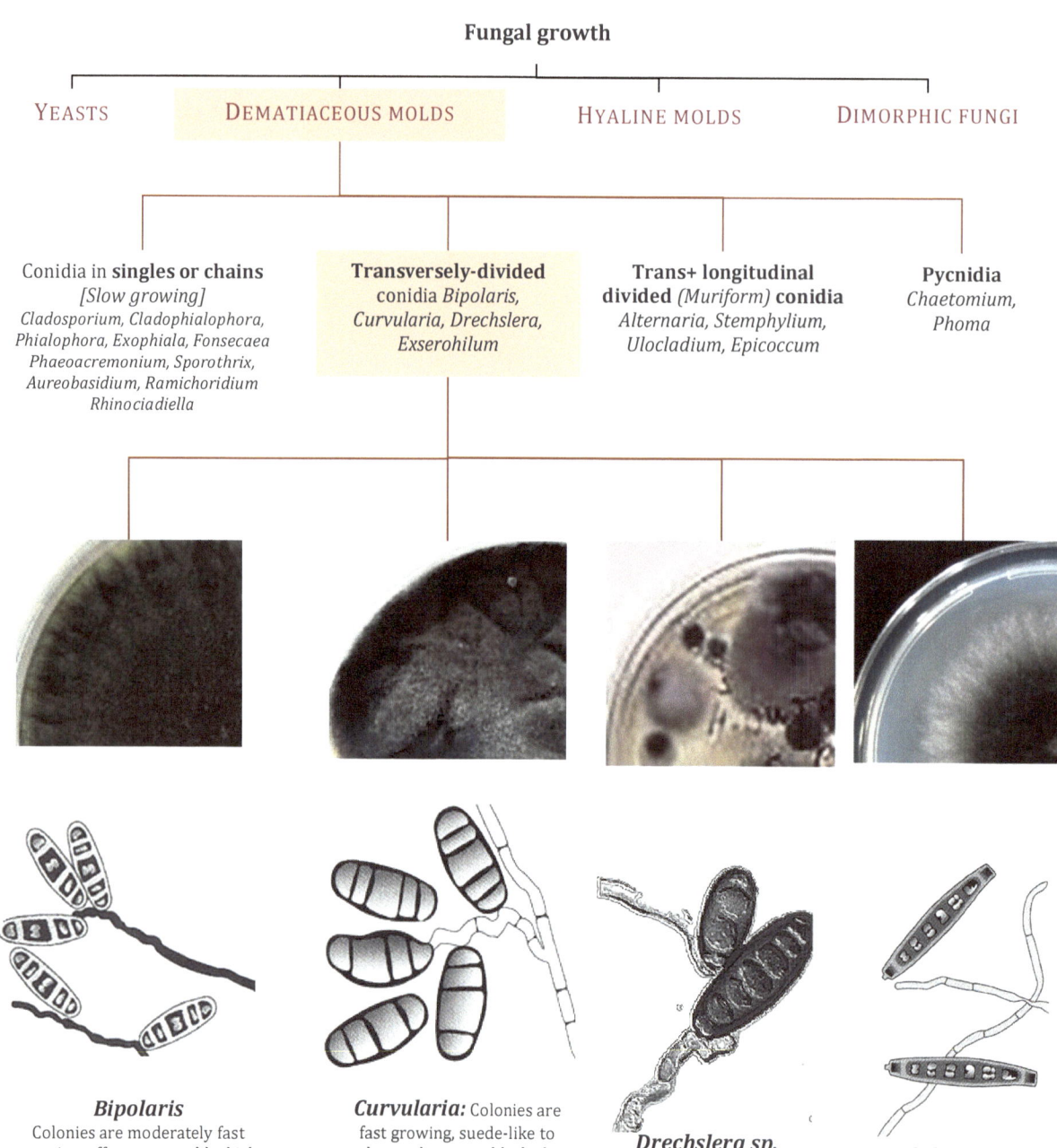

Bipolaris
Colonies are moderately fast growing, effuse, grey to blackish brown, suede-like to floccose with a black reverse.
Microscopy: shows sympodial development of **pale brown** pigmented, pseudoseptate conidia on a geniculate or zig-zag rachis. Conidia are produced through pores in the conidiophore wall (poroconidia) and are straight, fusiform to ellipsoidal, rounded at both ends, smooth to finely roughened and germinating only from the ends

Curvularia: Colonies are fast growing, suede-like to downy, brown to blackish brown with a black reverse.
Microscopy: Conidia are **pale brown**, with three or more **transverse septa** and are formed apically through a pore (poroconidia) in a sympodially elongating geniculate conidiophore similar to *Drechslera*. Conidia are cylindrical or slightly curved, with one of the central cells being larger and darker. Germination is bipolar and some species may have a prominent hilum

Drechslera sp.
Colonies are fast growing, suede-like to downy, brown to blackish brown with a black reverse.
Microcopy: Conidia are **pale to dark brown**, usually cylindrical, straight, smooth-walled, and are formed apically in a sympodially elongating geniculate conidiophore. Conidia are **transversely septate** with the septum delimiting the basal cell formed first during conidium maturation

Exserohilum: Colonies are grey to blackish-brown, suede-like to floccose in texture, olivaceous black reverse.
Microscopy: Conidia are straight, curved or slightly bent, ellipsoidal to fusiform and are formed apically through a pore on a sympodially elongating geniculate conidiophore. Conidia have a strongly protruding, truncate hilum and the septum above the hilum is usually thickened and dark

Fungal growth

- YEASTS
- DEMATIACEOUS MOLDS
- HYALINE MOLDS
- DIMORPHIC FUNGI

Dematiaceous molds

- **Conidia in singles or chains** [Slow growing]
  Cladosporium, Cladophialophora, Phialophora, Exophiala, Fonsecaea Phaeoacremonium, Sporothrix, Aureobasidium, Ramichoridium Rhinociadiella
- **Transversely-divided conidia** *Bipolaris, Curvularia, Drechslera, Exserohilum*
- **Trans+ longitudinal divided (Muriform) conidia** *Alternaria, Ulocladium, Epicoccum, and Stemphylium, Pithomyces*
- **Pycnidia** *Chaetomium, Phoma*

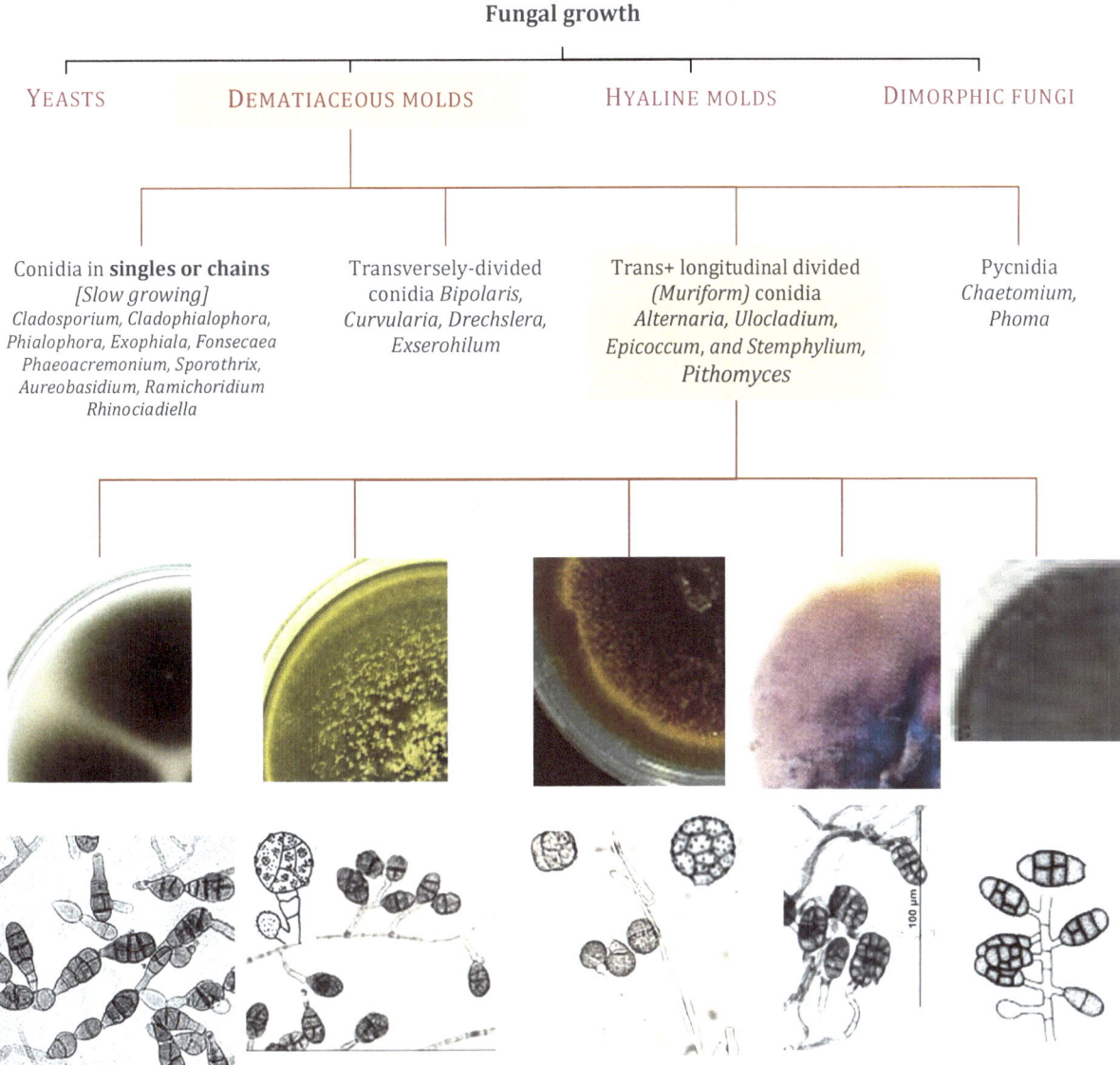

Alternaria alternate: Colonies are fast growing, black to olivaceous-black or greyish, and are suede-like to floccose. Microscopy: branched acropetal chains of multicelled conidia are produced sympodially sometimes branched, short or elongate conidiophores. Conidia are obclavate, obpyriform, sometimes ovoid or ellipsoidal, often with a short conical or cylindrical beak, pale brown, smooth-walled or verrucose

Ulocladium: Colonies are rapid growing, brown to olivaceous-black or greyish and suede-like to floccose. Microscopy: numerous, usually solitary, multicelled conidia (dictyoconidia) are formed through a pore (poroconidia) by a sympodially elongating geniculate conidiophore. Conidia are typically obovoid (narrowest at the base), dark brown and often rough-walled. Seven species have been described all being saprophytes

Epicoccum: Colonies are fast growing, suede-like to downy, yellow to orange-brown diffusable pigmentation. Microscopy: Numerous black sporodochia are visible. Conidia are formed singly on conidiophores. Conidia are globose pyriform with a funnel-shaped base and broad attachment scar, often split with a protuberant basal cell. Conidia become multicellular, darkly pigmented and have verrucose external surface

Stemphylium: Colonies are rapid growing, brown to olivaceous-black or greyish and suede-like to floccose. Microscopy: solitary, darkly pigmented, terminal, multicellular conidia are formed on a distinctive conidiophore with a darker terminal swelling

Pithomyces: Colonies are fast growing, dark grey to black, suede-like to downy and produce darkly pigmented. Microscopy: multicellular conidia formed on small peg-like branches of the vegetative hyphae. Conidia are broadly elliptical, pyriform, and oblong

Fungal growth

- YEASTS
- DEMATIACEOUS MOLDS
- **HYALINE MOLDS**
- DIMORPHIC FUNGI

On SDA after 3-5 days → Mold growth with borders, pastel on surface, apron growth on periphery

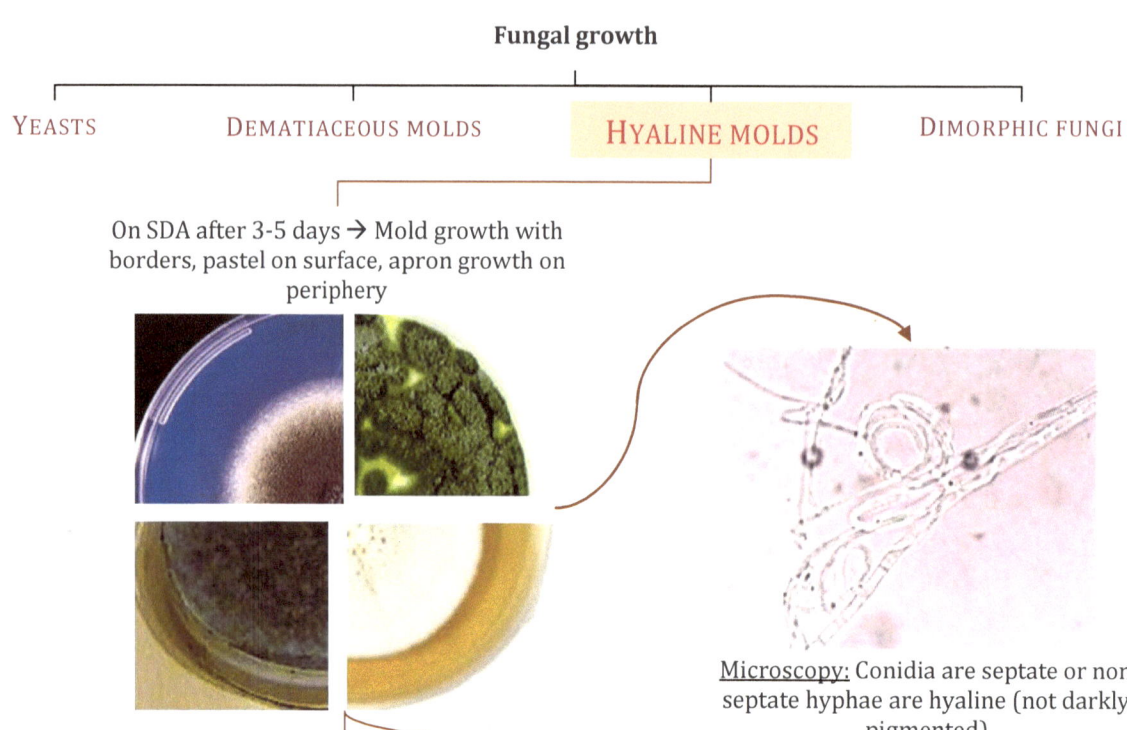

Microscopy: Conidia are septate or non septate hyphae are hyaline (not darkly pigmented)

SEPTATE HYALINE HYPHAE

HYALINE HYPHOMYCETES
In hyaline hyphomycetes fungi conidia **are not darkly pigmented**, colonies may be colorless or brightly colored. These include the agents of hyalohyphomycosis, Aspergillosis, and the dimorphic pathogens, like *Histoplasma capsulatum*

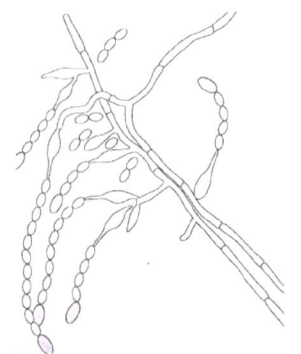

DERMATOPHYTES
Culture surface texture, topography and pigmentation are variable and are therefore the least reliable criteria for identification. Micro and/or macroconidia is the most reliable identification

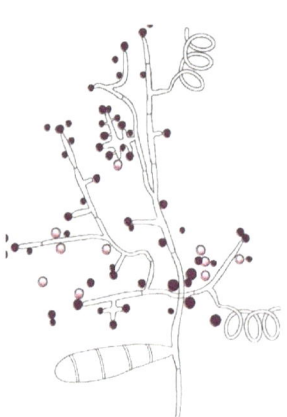

ASEPTATE HYALINE HYPHAE ZYGOMYCETES
Zygomycetes [BLACK BREAD MOLDS] are usually fast growing fungi [3 days 30°C → woolly filling Petri dish→ speckled. Microscopy: → Broad hyaline aseptate hyphae] characterized by primitive coenocytic (mostly aseptate) hyphae. Identification is based primarily on sporangial

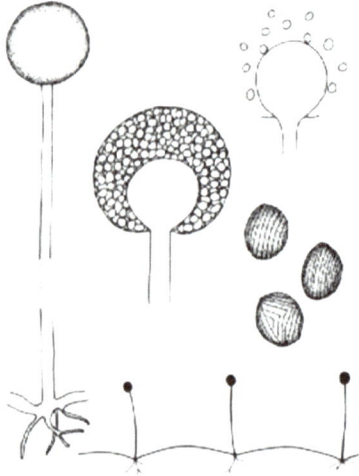

```
Fungal growth
├── YEASTS
├── DEMATIACEOUS MOLDS
├── HYALINE MOLDS
│    ├── SEPTATE HYALINE HYPHAE
│    │    ├── HYALINE HYPHOMYCETES
│    │    └── DERMATOPHYTES
│    └── ASEPTATE HYALINE HYPHAE
│         ZYGOMYCETES
│         ├── Rhizoids
│         │   Rhizopus, Mycocladus (Absidia);
│         │   Mortierella; Saksenaea
│         ├── No Rhizoids
│         │   Mucor, Syncephalastrum,
│         │   Cunninghamella
│         └── No rhizoid/ Yeast-like colonies
│             Basidiobolus, Conidiobolus
└── DIMORPHIC FUNGI
```

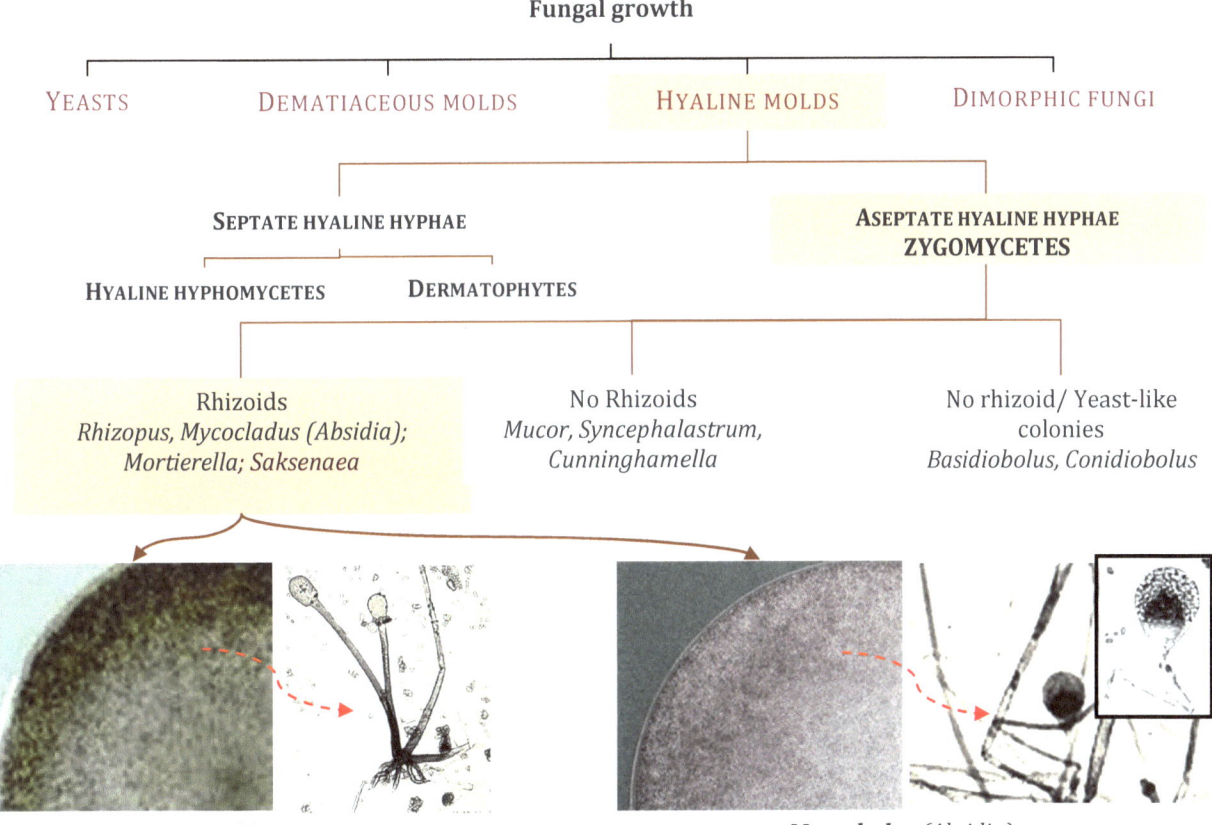

Rhizopus
Colonies *(Rhizopus oryzae)* are fast growing and cover an agar surface with a dense cottony growth that is at first white becoming grey or yellowish brown with sporulation *Rhizopus* is characterized by the presence of **stolons** and pigmented **rhizoids**, the formation of sporangiophores singly or in groups from nodes directly above the rhizoids, and apophysate, columellate, multi-spored, generally globose sporangia. After spore release the apophyses and columella often collapse to form an umbrella-like structure. Sporangiospores are globose to ovoid, one-celled, hyaline to brown and striate in many species

Mycocladus (Absidia)
Mycocladus corymbifera grows rapidly. The rapid growing, flat, woolly to cottony, and olive gray colonies mature within 4 days. The reverse side is uncolored and there is no pigment production. <u>Microscopy:</u> Hyphae differentiate into arched stolons bearing more or less verticillate sporangiophores at the internode, and rhizoids formed at the point of contact with the substrate. This feature separates species of *Mycocladus* from the genus Rhizopus, where the sporangia arise from the nodes and are therefore found opposite the rhizoids. The sporangia are relatively small, globose, pyriform- or **pear-shaped** and are supported by a characteristic funnel-shaped apophysis.

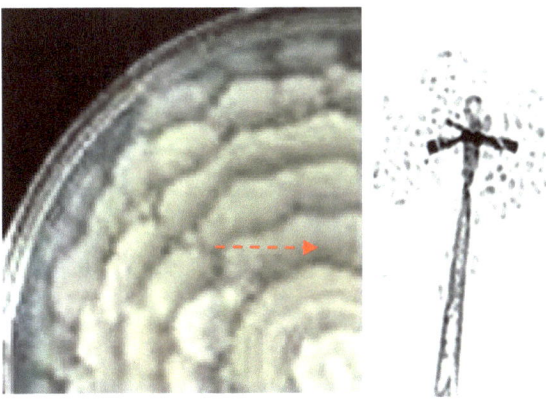

Mortierella
Fast growing, white to greyish white, downy, often with a broadly zonate or lobed (rosette-like) surface appearance and no reverse pigment. <u>Microscopy:</u> Sporangiophores are erect, wide at the base, arising from rhizoids and terminating with a compact cluster of short acrotonous (terminal) branches with many sporangia

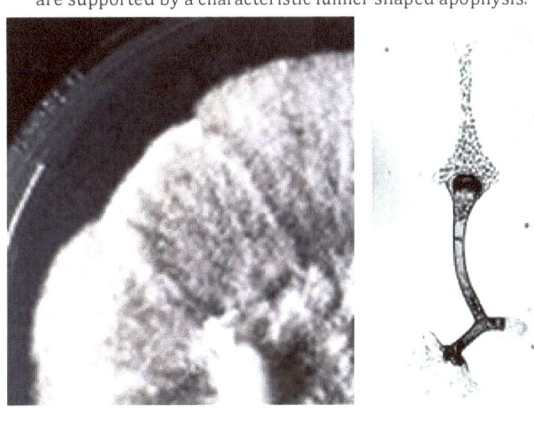

Saksenaea
Saksenaea vasiformis is fast growing, downy cottony, white with no reverse pigment. <u>Microscopy:</u> forms unique flask-shaped sporangia with columellae and simple, darkly pigmented rhizoids broad, non-septate hyphae.

Fungal growth

- **YEASTS**
- **DEMATIACEOUS MOLDS**
- **HYALINE MOLDS**
- **DIMORPHIC FUNGI**

HYALINE MOLDS

- **SEPTATE HYALINE HYPHAE**
  - **HYALINE HYPHOMYCETES**
  - **DERMATOPHYTES**
- **ASEPTATE HYALINE HYPHAE — ZYGOMYCETES**

Rhizoids
Rhizopus, Mycocladus (Absidia)

No Rhizoids
Mucor, Syncephalestrum, Saksenaea, Cunninghamella, Mortierella

No rhizoid / Yeast-like colonies
Basidiobolus, Conidiobolus

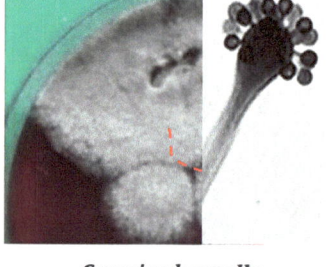

Mucor
Mucor can be differentiated from Absidia, Rhizomucor and Rhizopus by the absence of stolons and rhizoids. Colonies are very fast growing, cottony to fluffy, white to yellow, becoming dark-grey, with the development of sporangia. <u>Microscopy</u>: Sporangiophores are erect, simple or branched, forming large, terminal, and globose to spherical, multispored sporangia, without apophyses and with well-developed subtending columellae. Sporangiospores are hyaline, grey or brownish, globose to ellipsoidal, and smooth-walled or finely ornamented. Chlamydospores and zygospores may also be present.

Cunninghamella
Cunninghamella: fast growing, white at first, but becoming rather dark grey and powdery with development. <u>Microscopy</u>: Sporangiophores up to 20 um wide, straight, with verticillate or solitary branches. Vesicles subglobose to pyriform. Sporangiola are globose, ellipsoidal, verrucose or short-echinulate, hyaline singly but brownish in mass.

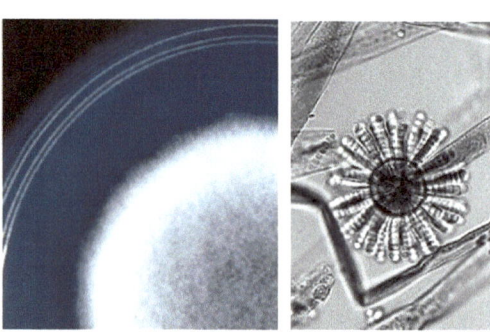

Syncephalastrum
Syncephalastrum racemosum: Fast growing, cottony to fluffy, white to light grey, becoming dark grey with the development of sporangia. <u>Microscopy</u>: producing sympodially branching sporangiophores with terminal vesicles bearing merosporangia.

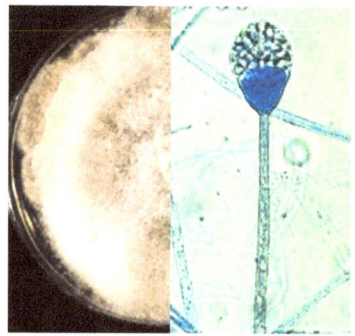

Apophysomyces elegans
Colonies are fast growing, white becoming creamy white to buff with age, downy with no reverse pigment, and are composed of broad, sparsely septate (coenocytic) hyphae typical of a zygomycetous fungus.

Fungal growth

- YEASTS
- DEMATIACEOUS MOLDS
- HYALINE MOLDS
- DIMORPHIC FUNGI

Hyaline molds

Septate hyaline hyphae
- Hyaline hyphomycetes
- Dermatophytes

Aseptate hyaline hyphae — ZYGOMYCETES

- **Rhizoids**: *Rhizopus, Absidia*
- **No Rhizoids**: *Mucor, Syncephalestrum, Saksenaea, Cunninghamella, Mortierella*
- **No rhizoid / Yeast-like colonies**: *Basidiobolus, Conidiobolus*

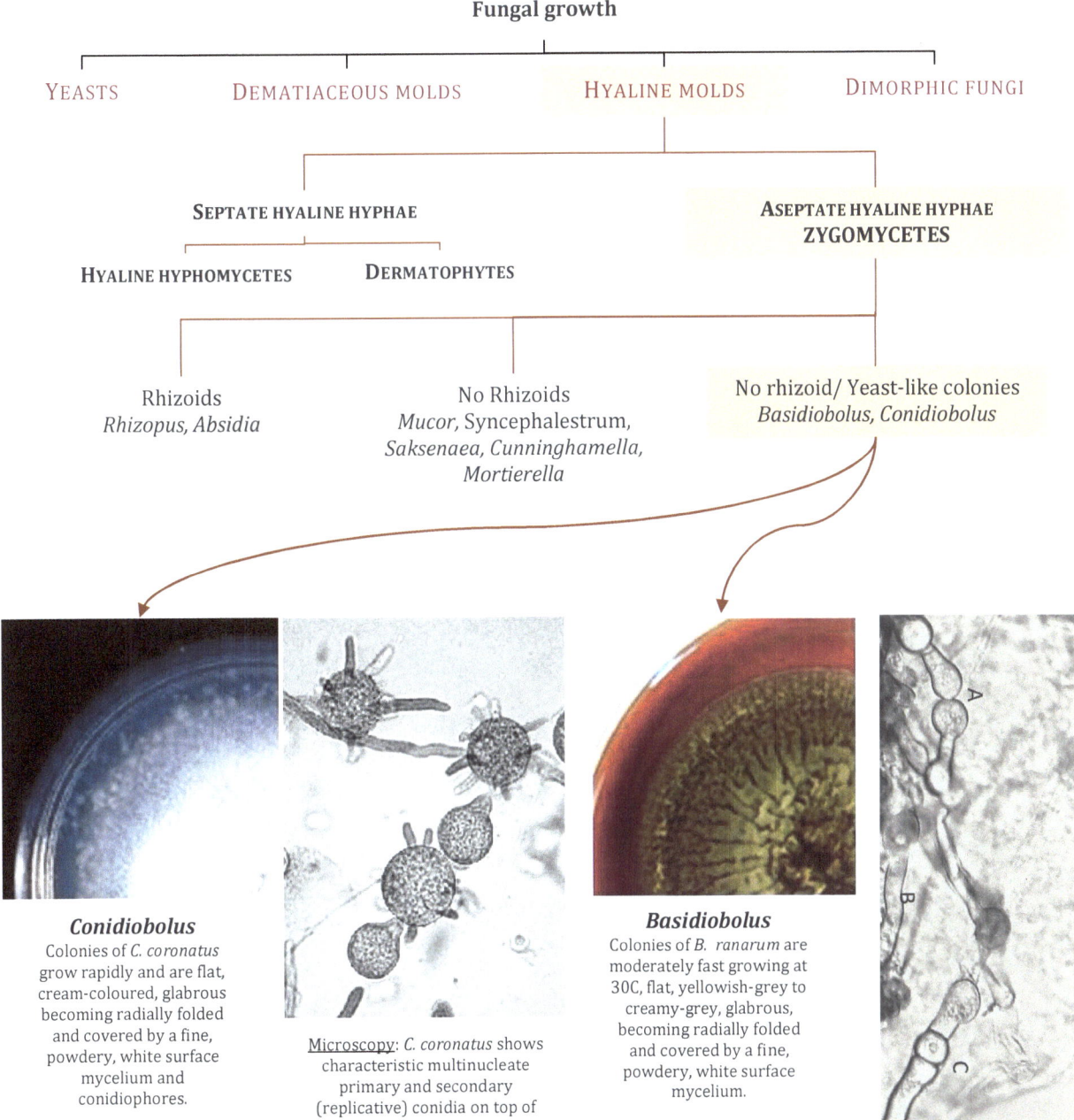

Conidiobolus
Colonies of *C. coronatus* grow rapidly and are flat, cream-coloured, glabrous becoming radially folded and covered by a fine, powdery, white surface mycelium and conidiophores.

Microscopy: *C. coronatus* shows characteristic multinucleate primary and secondary (replicative) conidia on top of unbranched conidiophores. Each subspherical conidium is discharged as a result of the pressure developed within the conidium, and each bears a more or less prominent papilla after discharge. Conidia may also produce hair-like appendages, called villae

Basidiobolus
Colonies of *B. ranarum* are moderately fast growing at 30C, flat, yellowish-grey to creamy-grey, glabrous, becoming radially folded and covered by a fine, powdery, white surface mycelium.

B. ranarum are produces sexual reproduction characteristic for zygomycetes. Note the broad hyaline hyphae which induced zygophores (B) bearing protuberances globose one-celled conidia. Two zygophores (A) to form zygospores (C).

Fungal growth

- **YEASTS**
- **DEMATIACEOUS MOLDS**
- **HYALINE MOLDS**
- **DIMORPHIC FUNGI**

Hyaline molds

- **SEPTATE HYALINE HYPHAE**
- **ASEPTATE HYALINE HYPHAE — ZYGOMYCETES**

Septate hyaline hyphae

- **HYALINE HYPHOMYCETES**
- **DERMATOPHYTES**

Dermatophytes

- *Trichophyton*
- *Microsporum*
- *Epidermophyton*

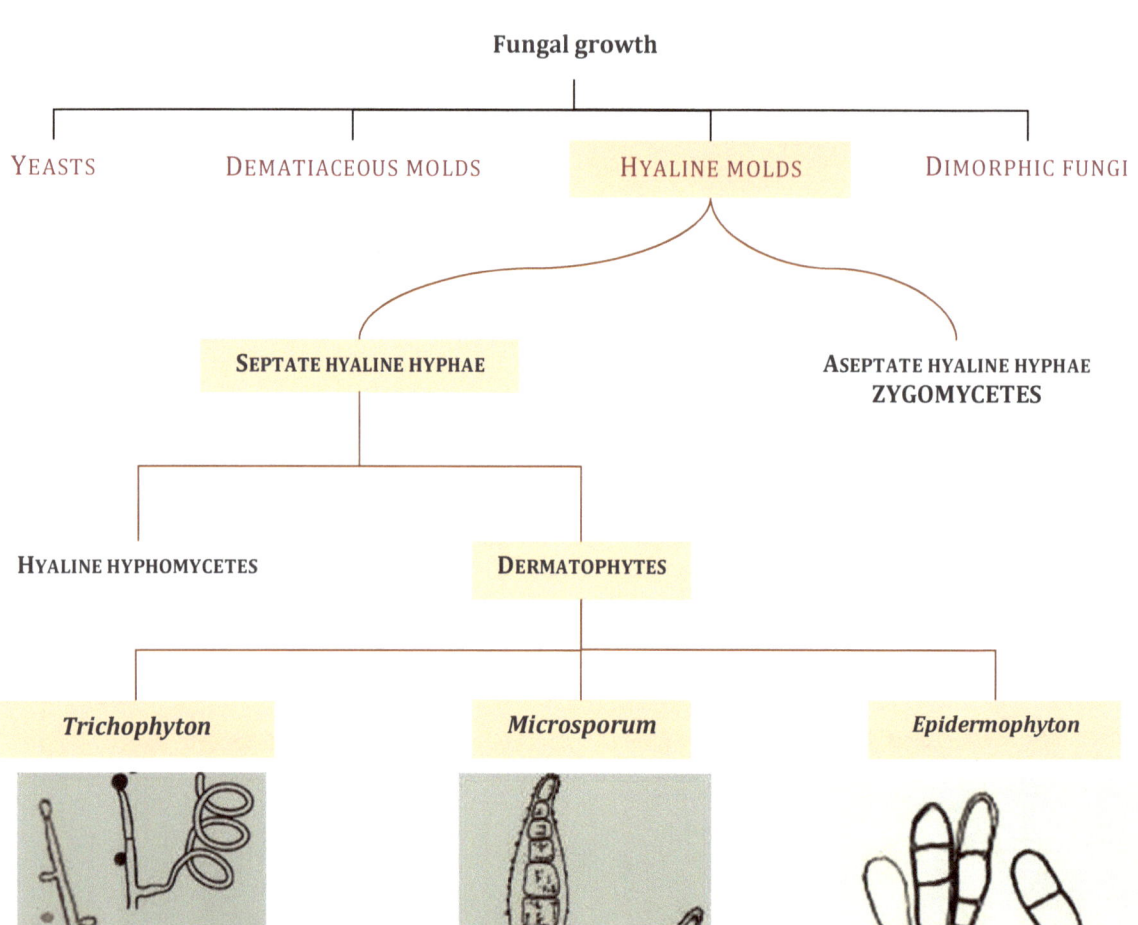

Colonies of the genus *Trichophyton* are variable and least reliable criteria for identification generally flat, spreading granular, with a deep cream to buff to pale cinnamon coloured. Microscopy: characterized by presence of both macro- and microconidia borne laterally directly on the hyphae or on short pedicels, and are clavate to fusiform (**cigar shape**), and range from 4 to 8 by 8 to 50 um in size. Macroconidia are few or absent in many species.

Colonies of the genus *Microsporum* are usually flat, spreading, suede-like to granular, with a deep cream to tawny-buff to pale cinnamon coloured red surface. Many cultures develop a central white downy dome or a fluffy white tuft of mycelium and some also have a narrow white peripheral boarder. Microscopy: characterized by presence of both macro- and microconidia on short conidiophores. Macroconidia are hyaline, multiseptate, variable in form, fusiform, **spindle-shaped** to obovate, ranging from 7 to 20 by 30 to 160 um in size

Colonies of the genus *Epidermophyton* are usually slow growing, greenish-brown or khaki coloured with a suede-like surface, raised and folded in the centre, with a flat periphery and submerged fringe of growth. Older cultures may develop white pleomorphic tufts of mycelium. A deep yellowish-brown reverse pigment is usually present. Microscopy: shows characteristic smooth, thin-walled macroconidia which are often produced in clusters growing directly from the hyphae (**club shape**). Numerous chlamydoconidia are formed in older cultures. No microconidia are formed.

Fungal growth

- YEASTS
- DEMATIACEOUS MOLDS
- HYALINE MOLDS
  - SEPTATE HYALINE HYPHAE
    - HYALINE HYPHOMYCETES
    - DERMATOPHYTES
      - *Trichophyton*
      - *Microsporum*
      - *Epidermophyton*
  - ASEPTATE HYALINE HYPHAE
    ZYGOMYCETES
- DIMORPHIC FUNGI

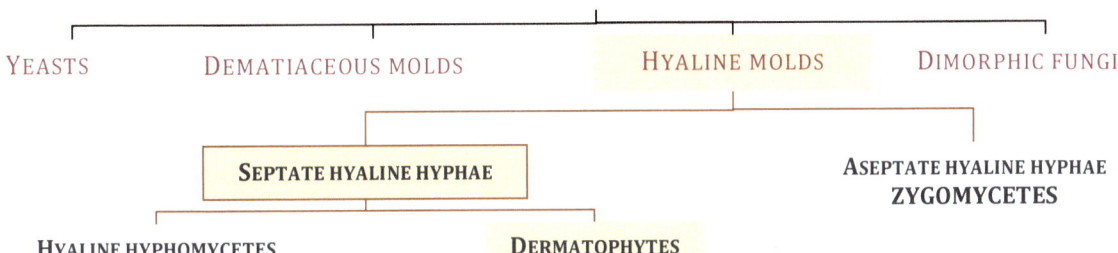

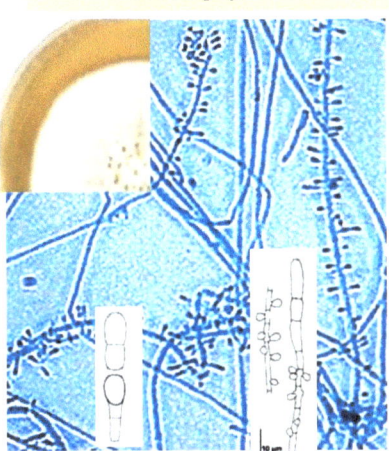

Trich. rubrum Growth rate: slow to moderately rapid. Texture: downy to cottony. Thallus color: white to pale pink. Reverse: blood red (PDA) to reddish brown (SDA, Mycosel). few pyriform, lateral microconidia pencil shaped macroconidia uncommon microconidia form on macroconidia arthroconidia produced from hyphae and macroconidia

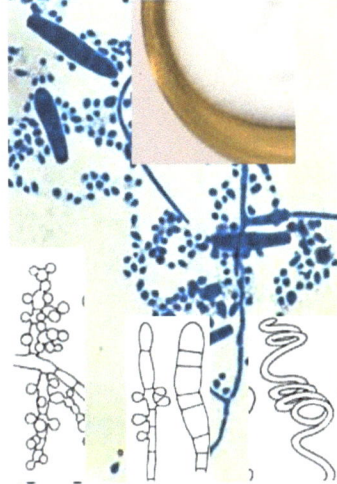

Trich. mentagrophyte: anthrophilic and zoophilic, worldwide, feet, body, nails, beard, scalp, hand, groin, Growth moderate → Granular or Velvety buff to tan Reverse: pale yellow, tan, or reddish brown →→ round microconidia in grape-like clusters, spiral hyphae +/- cigar shaped, Urease+; Hair perforation + hyphomycetes (Line molds)

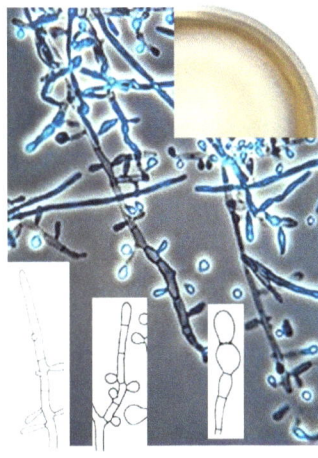

Trich. tonsurans: anthrophilic, worldwide, scalp, body "shower sites", occasionally nails, Moderately fast → suede like with radial folds, white to creamy yellow, rose Reverse: lemon yellow →→ many pyriform microconidia on stalks, balloon forms rare, distorted macroconidia. May have *spiral* hyphae. Urease+; Hair perforation -

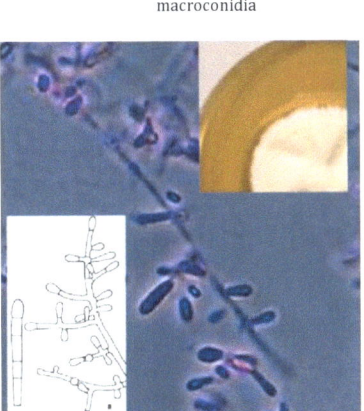

Trich. terrestre: geophilic, worldwide, nonpathogenic, moderately rapid → velvety to granular, flat to folded, white to yellow; Reverse yellow, Microconidia intergrade with macroconidia, transition forms microconidia pyriform to elongate, often on pedicels macroconidia have *chlamydospores*, spirals, raquet hyphae, Urease+; Hair perforation +

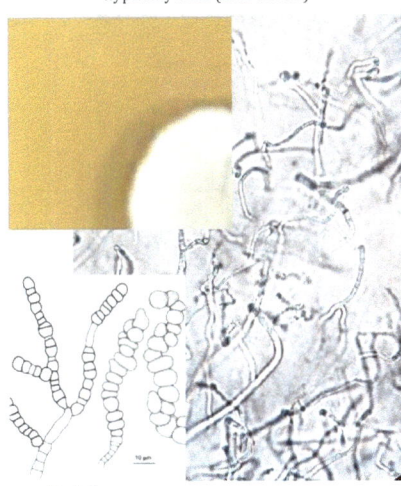

Trich. verrucosum: zoophilic, worldwide, scalp, beard, body, occasionally nails. Slow better at 35°C → waxy or glabrous heaped or flat, white, grey or yellow; reverse: colorless characteristic chains of chlamydospores at 35°C; Urease+; Hair perforation -

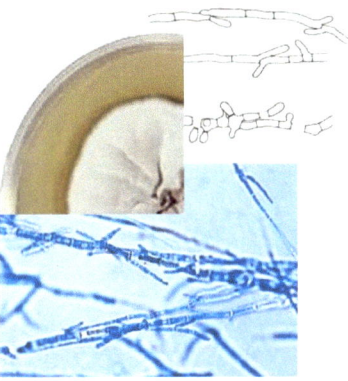

Trich. soudanense Growth rate is slow to moderately rapid and texture of colonies ranges from glabrous, with a filamentous fridge which surrounds the colony; and
Both surface and reverse colony color is pale yellow to rusty, red purple at times. Hyphae are observed with reflexive branching and are typically present; Microconidia are more or less present,

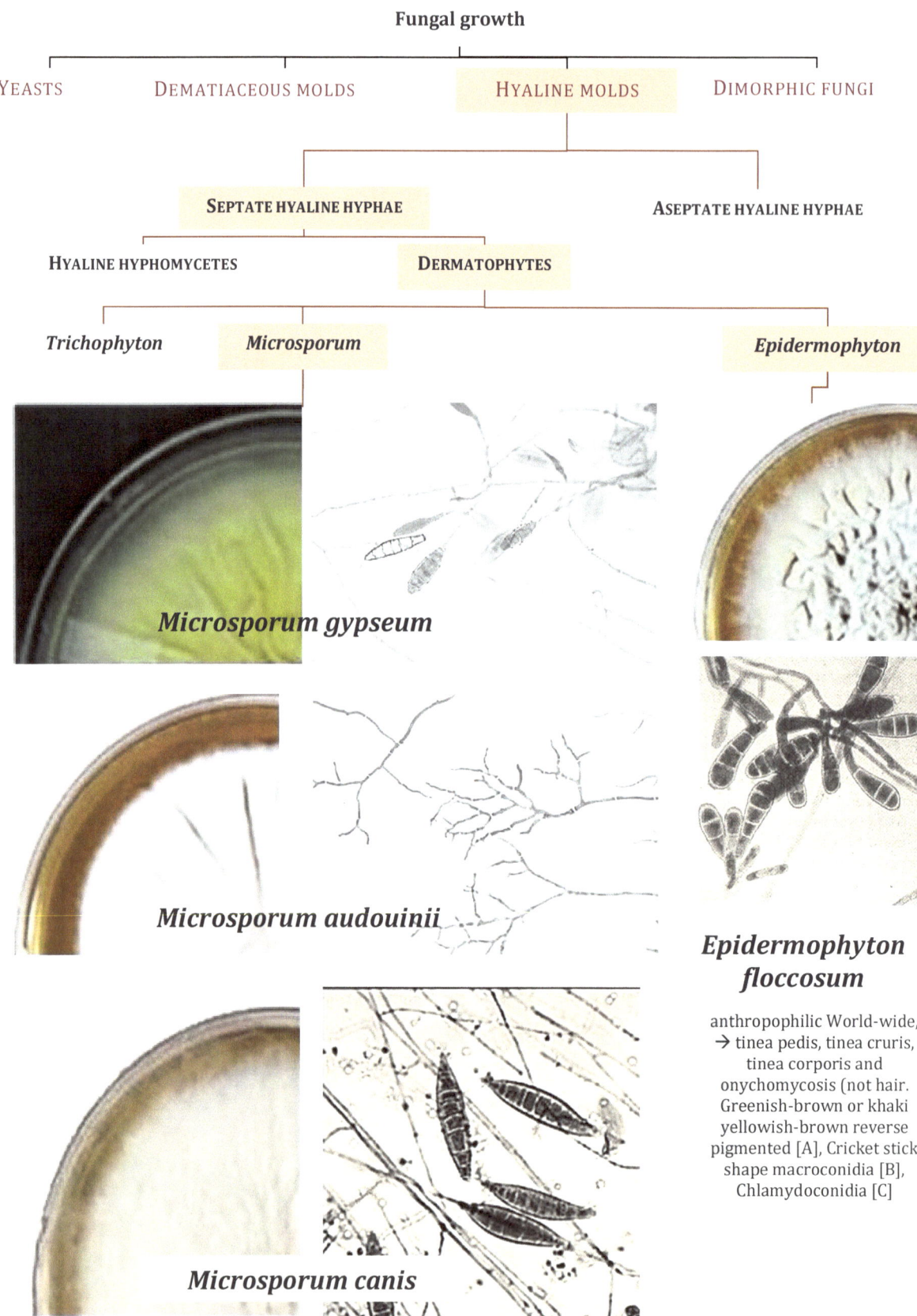

Epidermophyton floccosum

anthropophilic World-wide, → tinea pedis, tinea cruris, tinea corporis and onychomycosis (not hair. Greenish-brown or khaki yellowish-brown reverse pigmented [A], Cricket stick shape macroconidia [B], Chlamydoconidia [C]

Fungal growth

- YEASTS
- DEMATIACEOUS MOLDS
- HYALINE MOLDS
  - SEPTATE HYALINE HYPHAE
    - HYALINE HYPHOMYCETES
    - DERMATOPHYTES
  - ASEPTATE HYALINE HYPHAE
- DIMORPHIC FUNGI

On SDA after 3-5 days → Mold growth, borders, **pastel** on surface, **apron** growth on periphery Line molds

Conidia borne singly
Beauvaria, Blastomyces, Histoplasma, Sepedonium, Scedosporium

Conidia in chains
Madurella, Paecilomyces, Penicillium, Scopulariopsis

Conidia in cluster
Acremonium, Fusarium, Gliocladium, Trichoderma, Verticillium

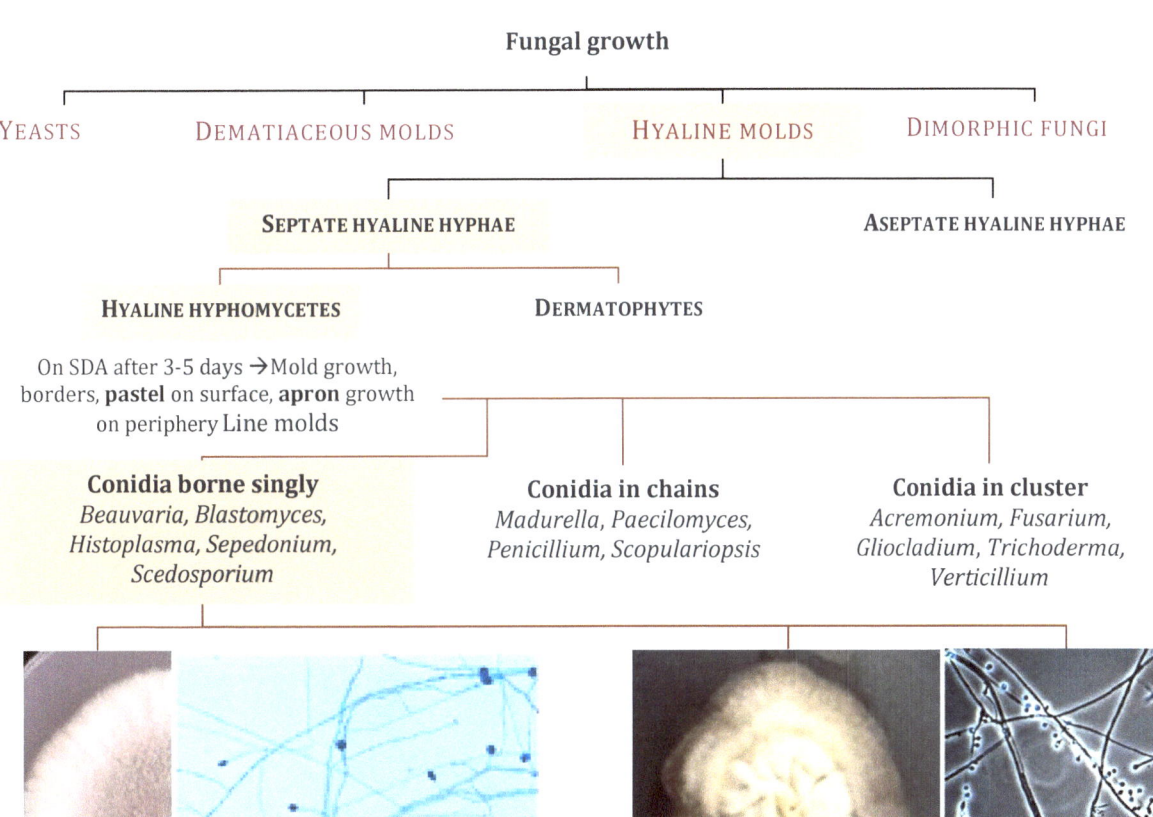

Scedosporium
Scedosporium apiospermum: Colonies are fast growing, greyish-white, suede-like to downy with a greyish-black reverse. Microscopy: Numerous **single-celled**, pale-brown, broadly clavate to ovoid conidia, rounded above with truncate bases are observed. Conidia are borne singly or in small groups on elongate, simple or branched conidiophores or laterally on hyphae

Mould form of *Blastomyces*
At 25C, colonies are variable in both morphology and rate of growth. They may grow rapidly, producing a fluffy white mycelium, or slowly as glabrous, tan, non-sporulating colonies. Growth and sporulation are enhanced by nitrogenous substances found in starling dung and yeast extract. Most strains become pleomorphic with age. Microscopy: hyaline, ovoid to pyriform, one-celled, conidia borne on short lateral or terminal hyphal branches

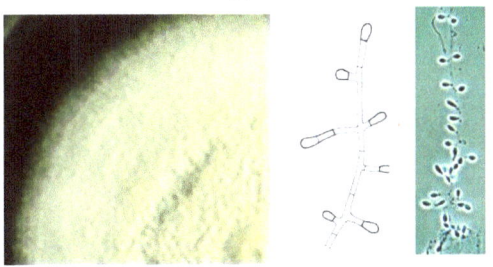

Chrysosporium
Chrysosporium tropicum: Colonies are moderately growing, flat, and white to tan to beige in colour, often with a powdery or granular surface texture. Reverse pigment absent or pale brownish-yellow with age. Microscopy: Hyaline, one-celled are produced directly on **vegetative** hyphae by non-specialized conidiogenous cells. Conidia are typically pyriform to clavate with truncate bases and are formed either intercalary (arthroconidia), laterally (often on pedicels) or terminally. No macroconidia or hyphal spirals are seen

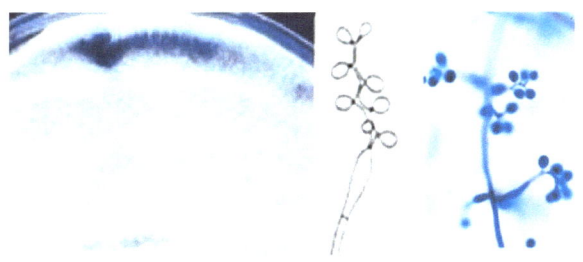

Beauveria
Beauvaria bassiana: Colonies are usually slow growing, downy, at first white but later often becoming yellow to pinkish. Microscopy: The genus Beauveria is characterized by the **sympodial** development of single-celled conidia on a geniculate or **zig-zag** rachis. Conidiogenous cells are flask-shaped, rachiform, proliferating sympodially and are often aggregated into sporodochia or synnemata. Conidia are hyaline and globose or ovoid in shape

Fungal growth

- YEASTS
- DEMATIACEOUS MOLDS
- **HYALINE MOLDS**
- DIMORPHIC FUNGI

HYALINE MOLDS

- **SEPTATE HYALINE HYPHAE**
- ASEPTATE HYALINE HYPHAE

SEPTATE HYALINE HYPHAE

- **HYALINE HYPHOMYCETES**
- DERMATOPHYTES

On SDA after 3-5 days → Mold growth, borders, **pastel** on surface, **apron** growth on periphery Line molds

Conidia borne singly	Conidia in chains	Conidia in cluster
Beauveria, Blastomyces, Histoplasma, Sepedonium, Scedosporium	*Madurella, Paecilomyces, Penicillium, Scopulariopsis*	*Acremonium, Fusarium, Gliocladium, Trichoderma, Verticillium*

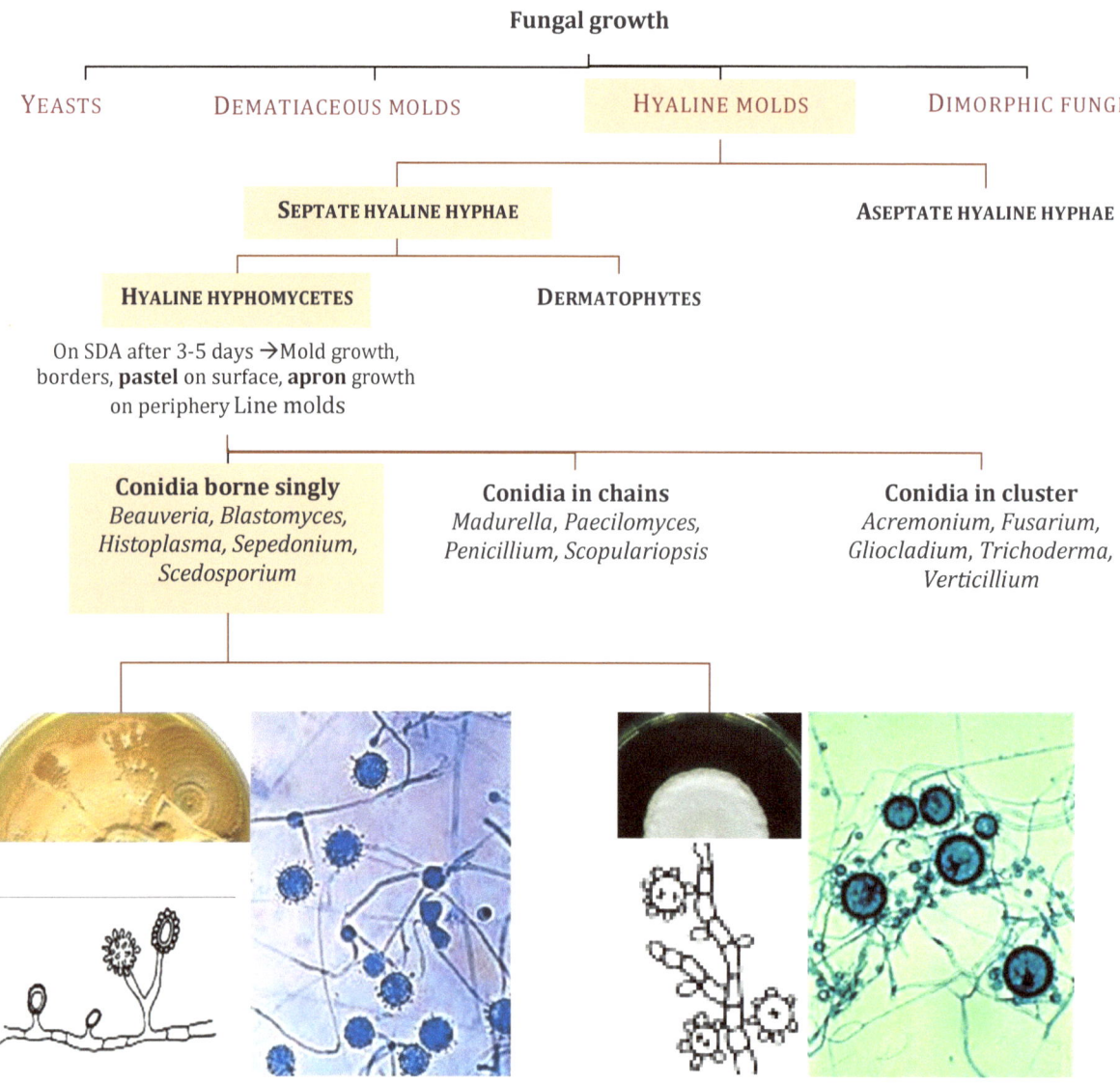

Sepedonium
Sepedonium sp.: Colonies are moderately fast growing, usually white to golden yellow, suede-like to downy, becoming fluffy with age. Microscopy: Conidiophores are hyaline, conidia are terminal, solitary, or in clusters, one-celled, globose to ovoid (tuberculate macroconidia), hyaline to amber, smooth to verrucose and usually with a thick wall. Resembles *Histoplasma* sp. In

Histoplasma (Mould form)
Histoplasma capsulatum exhibits thermal dimorphism by growing in living tissue or in culture at 37C as a budding yeast-like fungus or in soil or culture at temperatures below 30C as a mould. On SDA at 25C, colonies are slow growing, white or buff-brown, suede-like to cottony with a pale yellow-brown reverse. Other colony types are glabrous or verrucose, and a red pigmented strain has been noted.
Microscopy: shows the presence of characteristic large, rounded, single-celled, **tuberculate macroconidia** formed on short, hyaline, undifferentiated conidiophores. Microconidia, if present, are small, round to pyriform and borne on short branches or directly on the sides of the hyphae.

Fungal growth

- **YEASTS**
- **DEMATIACEOUS MOLDS**
- **HYALINE MOLDS**
  - **SEPTATE HYALINE HYPHAE**
    - **HYALINE HYPHOMYCETES**
      On SDA after 3-5 days → Mold growth, borders, **pastel** on surface, **apron** growth on periphery
      - **Conidia borne singly**
        Beauveria, Blastomyces, Histoplasma, Sepedonium, Scedosporium
      - **Conidia in chains**
        Madurella, Paecilomyces, Penicillium, Scopulariopsis
      - **Conidia in cluster**
        Acremonium, Fusarium, Gliocladium, Trichoderma, Verticillium
    - **DERMATOPHYTES**
  - **ASEPTATE HYALINE HYPHAE ZYGOMYCETES**
- **DIMORPHIC FUNGI**

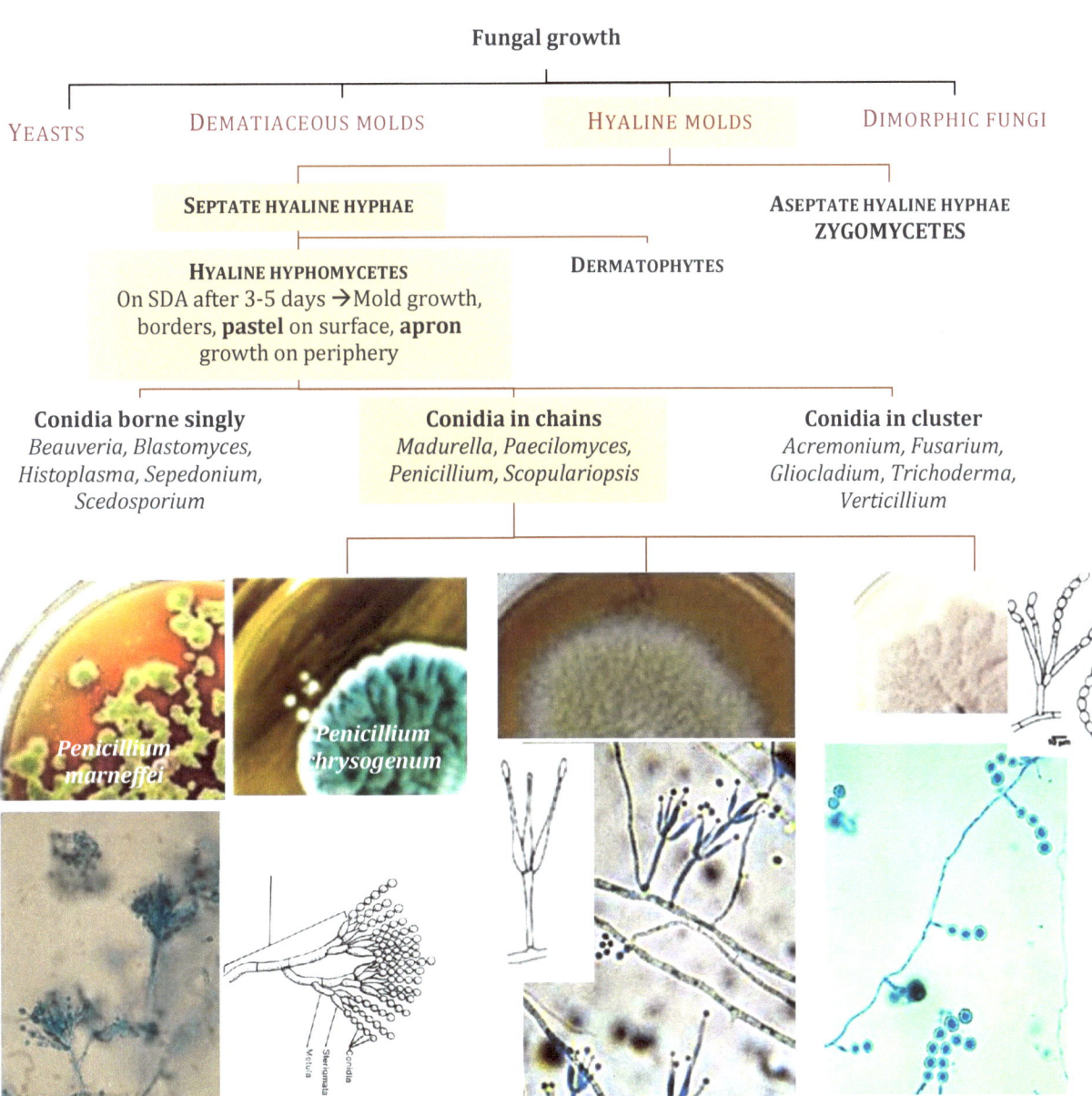

Penicillium
With only one exception, *P. marneffei*, which is thermally dimorphic), the members of the genus *Penicillium* are filamentous fungi. The colonies of *Penicillium* other than Penicillium marneffei are rapid growing, flat, filamentous, and velvety, woolly, or cottony in texture. The colonies are initially white and become blue green, gray green, olive gray, yellow or pinkish in time. P. marneffei is thermally dimorphic and produces filamentous, flat, radially sulcate colonies at 25°C. These colonies are bluish-gray-green at center and white at the periphery. The red, rapidly diffusing, soluble pigment observed from the reverse is very typical. At 37°C, *P. marneffei* colonies are cream to slightly pink in color and glabrous to convoluted in texture. Microscopy: septate hyaline hyphae, simple or branched conidiophores, metulae, phialides, and conidia are observed. In its filamentous phase, *P. marneffei* is microscopically similar to the other Penicillium species. In its yeast phase, on the other hand, *P. marneffei* is visualized as globose to elongated sausage-shaped cells

Paecilomyces
Paecilomyces: Colonies are fast growing, powdery or suede-like, gold, green-gold, yellow-brown, lilac or tan, but never green or blue-green as in Penicillium. Microscopy: have long slender divergent phialides. Phialides are swollen at their bases, gradually tapering into a rather long and slender neck, and occur solitarily, in pairs, as verticils, and in penicillate heads. Long, dry chains of single-celled, hyaline to dark, smooth or rough, ovoid to fusoid conidia are produced in basipetal succession from the phialides

Scopulariopsis
Colonies are fast growing, vary in color from white, cream, grey, buff to brown, black and are predominantly light brown. Microscopic morphology shows chains of single-celled conidia (ameroconidia) produced in basipetal succession by a specialized conidiogenous cell called an annellide. Once again, the term basocatenate can be used to describe such chains of conidia where the youngest conidium is at the basal end of the chain. In Scopulariopsis, annellides may be solitary, in groups, or organized into a distinct penicillus. Conidia are globose to pyriform, usually truncate, with a rounded distal portion, smooth to rough, and hyaline to brown in color.

Fungal growth

- **YEASTS**
- **DEMATIACEOUS MOLDS**
- **HYALINE MOLDS**
  - **SEPTATE HYALINE HYPHAE**
    - **HYALINE HYPHOMYCETES**
      On SDA after 3-5 days
      → Mold growth, borders, **pastel** on surface, **apron** growth on periphery
      - **Conidia borne singly**
        Beauveria, Blastomyces, Histoplasma, Sepedonium, Scedosporium
      - **Conidia in chains**
        Madurella, Paecilomyces, Penicillium, Scopulariopsis
      - **Conidia in cluster**
        Acremonium, Fusarium, Gliocladium, Trichoderma, Verticillium
    - **DERMATOPHYTES**
  - **ASEPTATE HYALINE HYPHAE**
    ZYGOMYCETES
- **DIMORPHIC FUNGI**

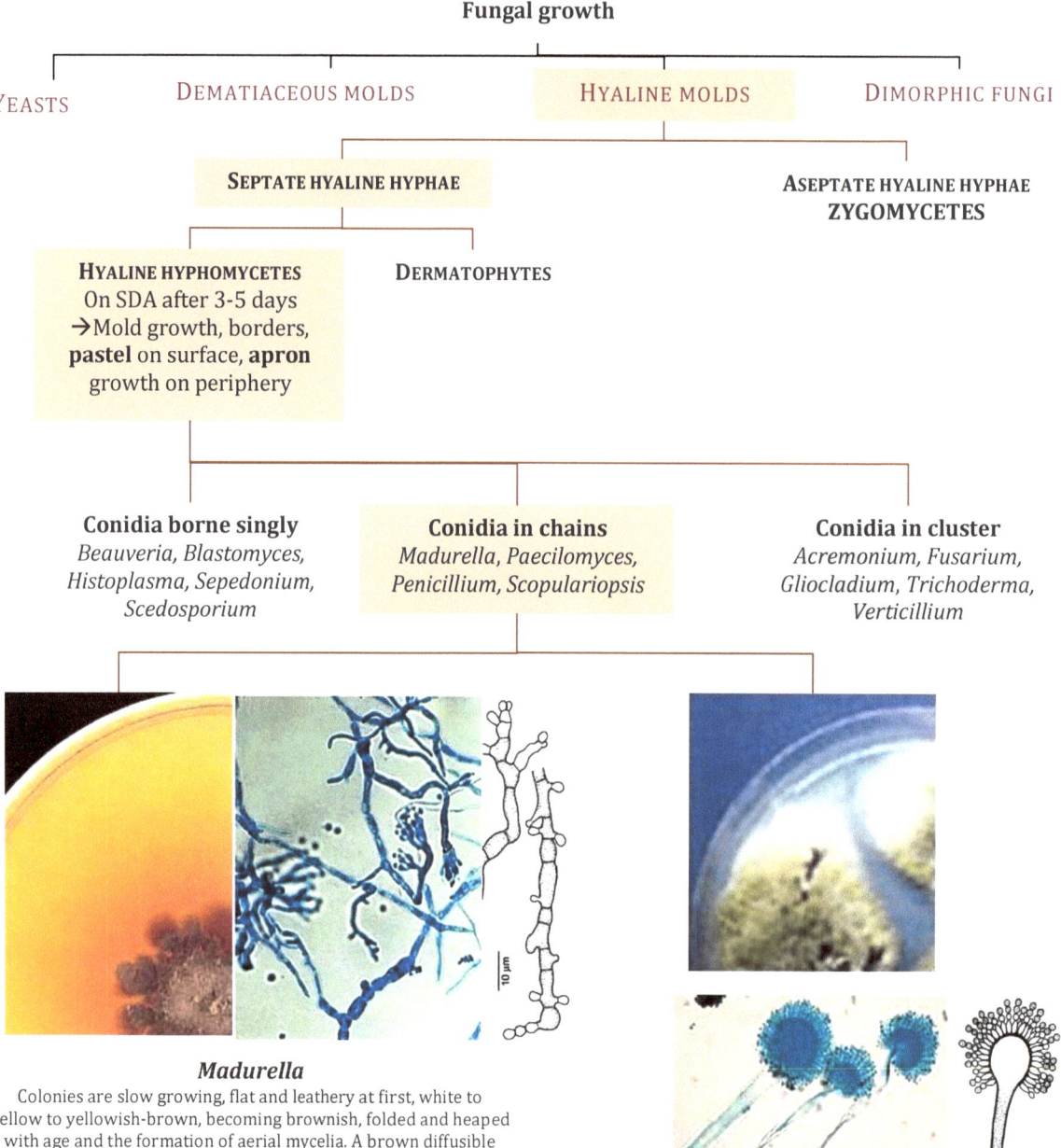

Madurella
Colonies are slow growing, flat and leathery at first, white to yellow to yellowish-brown, becoming brownish, folded and heaped with age and the formation of aerial mycelia. A brown diffusible pigment is characteristically produced in primary cultures.
Microscopy: Although most cultures are sterile, two types of conidiation have been observed, the first being flask-shaped phialides that bear rounded conidia, the second being simple or branched conidiophores bearing pyriform conidia (3-5 um) with truncated bases. The optimum temperature for growth of this mould is 37C.

Aspergillus
Aspergillus colonies are usually fast growing, white, yellow, yellow-brown, brown to black or shades of green, and they mostly consist of a dense felt of erect conidiophores. Microscopy: Conidiophores terminate in a vesicle covered with either a single palisade-like layer of phialides (uniseriate) or a layer of subtending cells (metulae) which bear small whorls of phialides (the so-called biseriate structure). The vesicle, phialides, metulae (if present) and conidia form the conidial head. Conidia are one-celled, smooth- or rough-walled, hyaline or pigmented and are basocatenate, forming long dry chains which may be divergent (radiate) or aggregated in compact columns (columnar). Some species may produce hülle cells or sclerotia.

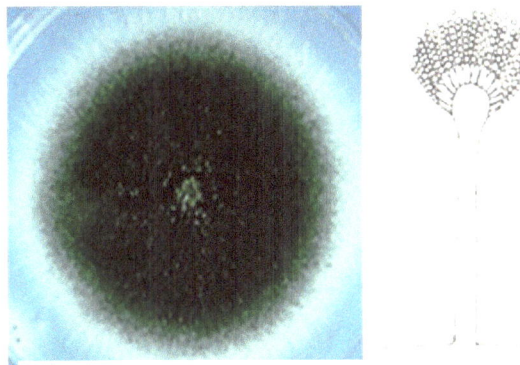 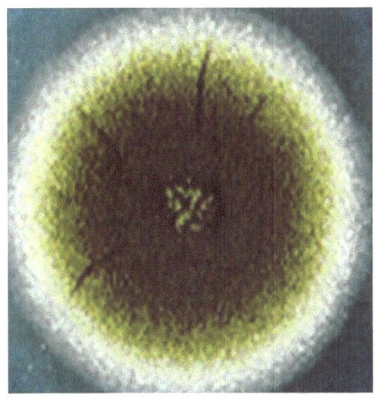 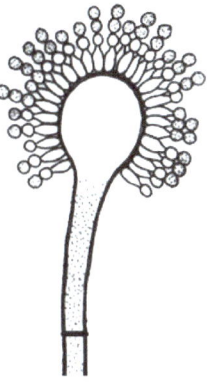

Aspergillus fumigatus
Blue-green surface pigmentation with a suede-like surface. Conidiophores are short, smooth-walled and have conical-shaped terminal vesicles, uniseriate row of phialides on the upper two thirds of the vesicle, green rough wall conidia

Aspergillus flavus
Granular, flat, often with radial grooves, yellow at first but quickly becoming bright to dark yellow-green with age. Conidial heads typically radiate with both uniseriate and biseriate. Pale green and conspicuously echinulate

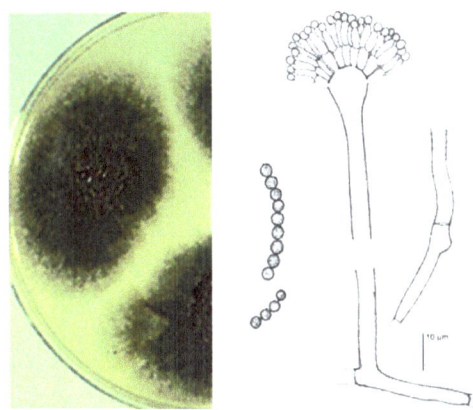 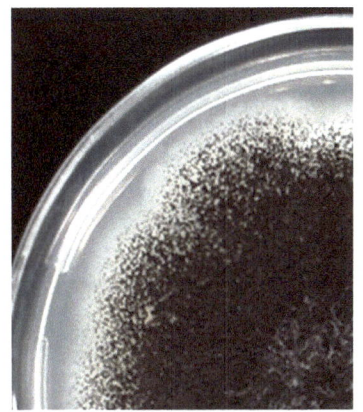 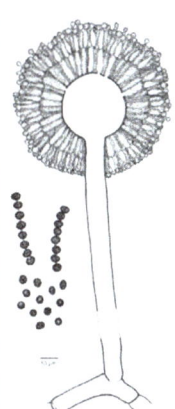

Aspergillus nidulans
Plain green in color with dark red-brown cleistothecia developing within and upon the conidial layer. Reverse may be olive to gray or purple-brown. conidial heads are short, columnar and biseriate, Conidia are globose (3.0-3.5 um in diameter) and rough-walled

Aspergillus niger
white or yellow basal felt covered by a dense layer of dark-brown to black conidial heads. Conidial heads are large (up to 3 mm x 15-20 um in diameter), globose, dark brown, becoming radiate and tending to split into several loose columns with age, Conidia are globose to subglobose (3.5-5.0 um in diameter), dark brown to black and rough-walled

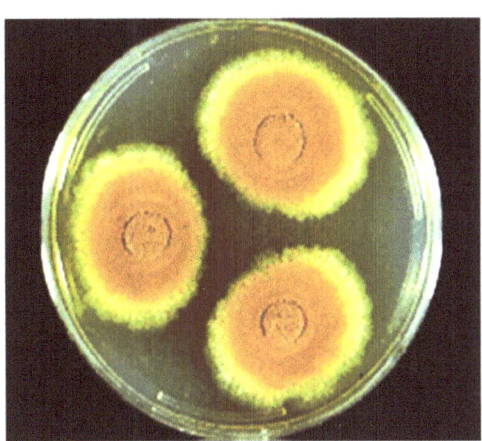 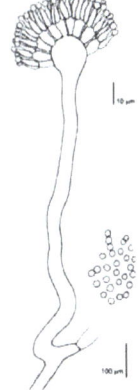

Aspergillus terreus
Granular, flat, often with radial grooves, yellow at first but quickly becoming bright to dark yellow-green with age. conidial heads are biseriate. , Conidia are globose to ellipsoidal (1.5-2.5 um in diameter), hyaline to slightly yellow and smooth-walled

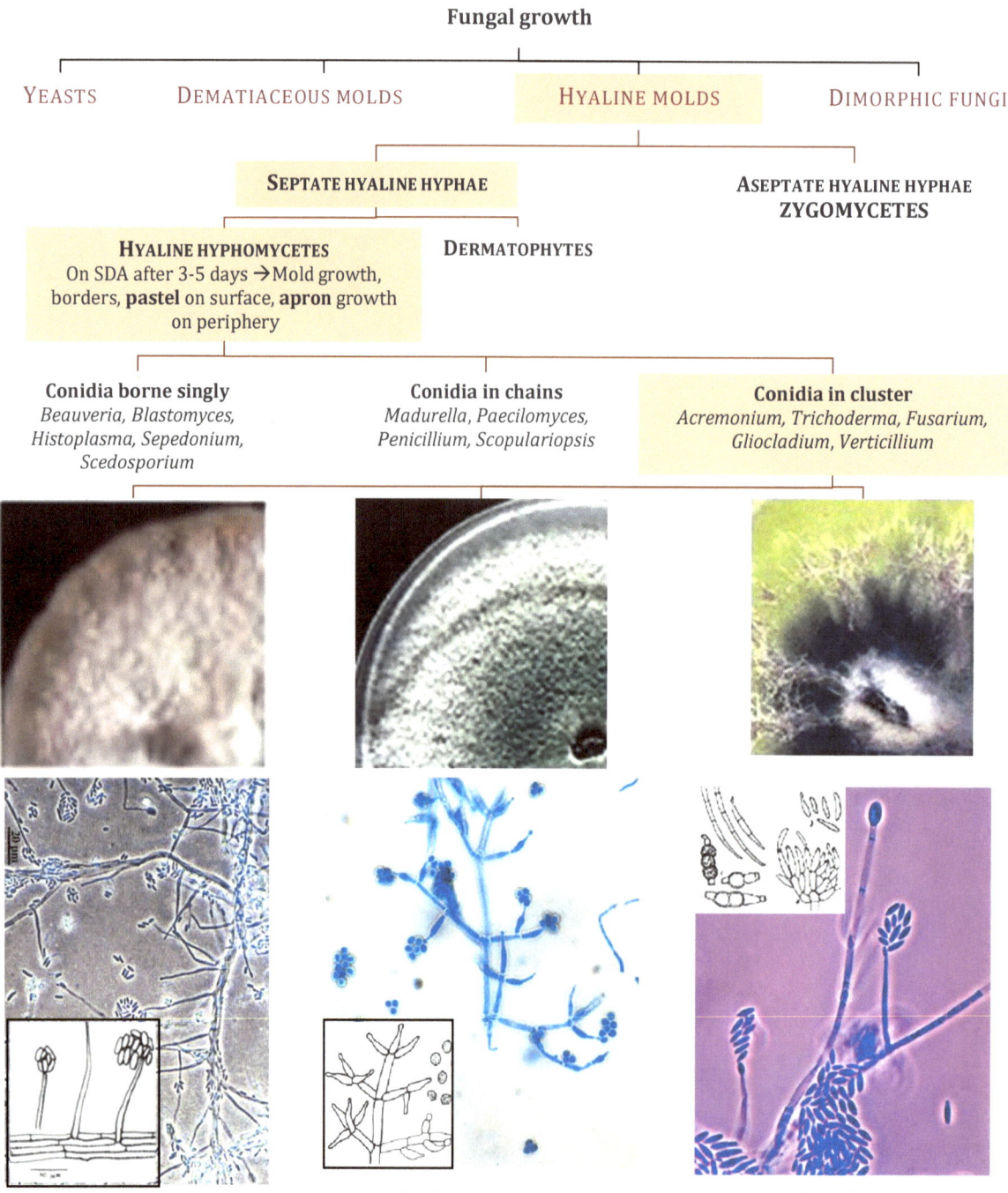

```
                          Fungal growth
        ┌──────────┬──────────────┬──────────────┬─────────────┐
    YEASTS   DEMATIACEOUS MOLDS   HYALINE MOLDS   DIMORPHIC FUNGI
                                        │
                          ┌─────────────┴─────────────┐
                   SEPTATE HYALINE HYPHAE     ASEPTATE HYALINE HYPHAE
                                                    ZYGOMYCETES
              ┌─────────────┬──────────┐
         HYALINE HYPHOMYCETES     DERMATOPHYTES
         On SDA after 3-5 days → Mold growth,
         borders, pastel on surface, apron growth
                     on periphery
```

Conidia borne singly	Conidia in chains	Conidia in cluster
Beauveria, Blastomyces, Histoplasma, Sepedonium, Scedosporium	*Madurella, Paecilomyces, Penicillium, Scopulariopsis*	*Acremonium, Trichoderma, Fusarium, Gliocladium, Verticillium*

Acremonium

Colonies are usually slow growing, often compact and moist at first, becoming powdery, suede-like or floccose with age, and may be white, grey, pink, rose or orange in color. <u>Microscopy:</u> Hyphae are fine and hyaline and produce mostly simple awl-shaped erect phialides. Conidia are usually one-celled, hyaline or pigmented, globose to cylindrical, and mostly aggregated in slimy heads at the apex of each phialide [**balls or chain**].

Trichoderma

Trichoderma harzianum: Colonies are fast growing, white and downy, later yellowish-green to deep green compact tufts, often only in small areas or in concentric ring-like zones on the agar surface. <u>Microscopy:</u> Conidiophores are repeatedly branched, irregularly verticillate, bearing clusters of divergent, often irregularly bent, flask-shaped phialides. Conidia are mostly green, sometimes hyaline, with smooth or rough walls and are formed in slimy conidial heads clustered at the tips of the phialides [inflated at the base]

Fusarium

F. oxysporum: Colonies are usually fast growing, pale or brightly colored (depending on the species) and may or may not have a cottony aerial mycelium. The color of the thallus varies from whitish to yellow, brownish, pink, reddish or lilac shades. <u>Microscopy:</u> Species of Fusarium typically produce both macro- and microconidia from slender phialides. Macroconidia are hyaline, two- to several-celled, fusiform- to sickle-shaped, mostly with an elongated apical cell and pedicellate basal cell. Microconidia are 1- to 2-celled, hyaline, pyriform, fusiform to ovoid (**sickle-shaped**), straight or curved. Chlamydoconidia may be present or absent

Fungal growth

- **YEASTS**
- **DEMATIACEOUS MOLDS**
- **HYALINE MOLDS**
  - **SEPTATE HYALINE HYPHAE**
    - **HYALINE HYPHOMYCETES**
      On SDA after 3-5 days
      → Mold growth, borders, **pastel** on surface, **apron** growth on periphery
    - **DERMATOPHYTES**
  - **ASEPTATE HYALINE HYPHAE** — ZYGOMYCETES
- **DIMORPHIC FUNGI**

Conidia borne singly
Beauveria, Blastomyces, Histoplasma, Sepedonium, Scedosporium

Conidia in chains
Madurella, Paecilomyces, Penicillium, Scopulariopsis

Conidia in cluster
Acremonium, Trichoderma, Fusarium, Gliocladium, Verticillium

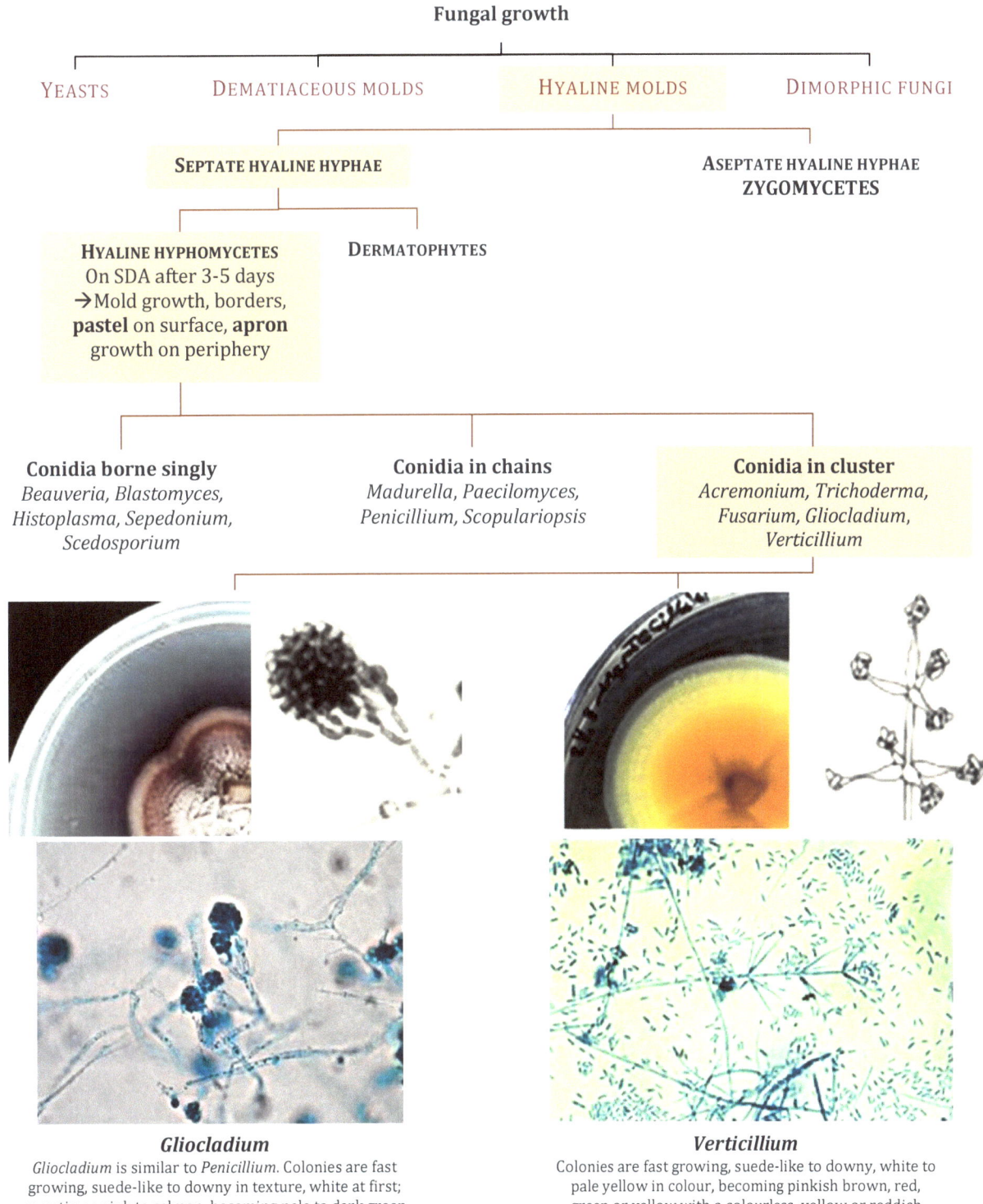

Gliocladium

Gliocladium is similar to *Penicillium*. Colonies are fast growing, suede-like to downy in texture, white at first; sometimes pink to salmon, becoming pale to dark green with sporulation. Microscopy: The most characteristic feature of the genus is the distinctive erect, often densely penicillate conidiophores with phialides which bear slimy, one-celled hyaline to green, smooth-walled conidia in heads or columns. Although, some penicillate conidiophores are always present, Gliocladium species may also produce verticillate branching conidiophores which can be confused with *Verticillium* or *Trichoderma*

Verticillium

Colonies are fast growing, suede-like to downy, white to pale yellow in colour, becoming pinkish brown, red, green or yellow with a colourless, yellow or reddish brown reverse. Microscopy: Conidiophores are usually well differentiated and erect, verticillately branched over most of their length, bearing whorls of slender awl-shaped divergent phialides. Conidia are hyaline or brightly coloured, mostly one-celled, and are usually borne in slimy heads

Fungal growth

- YEASTS
- DEMATIACEOUS MOLDS
- HYALINE MOLDS
- **DIMORPHIC FUNGI**

Dimorphic fungi are fungi which can exist as mold/ hyphal/ filamentous form (at room temperature 25°C) or as yeast (at body temperature 37°C)

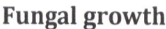

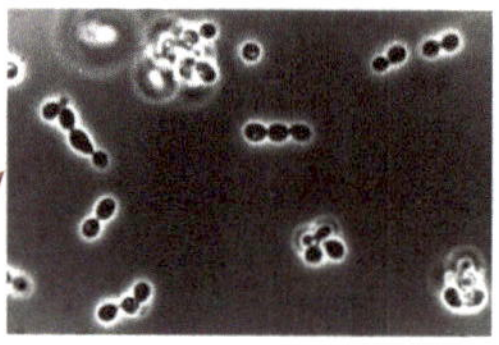

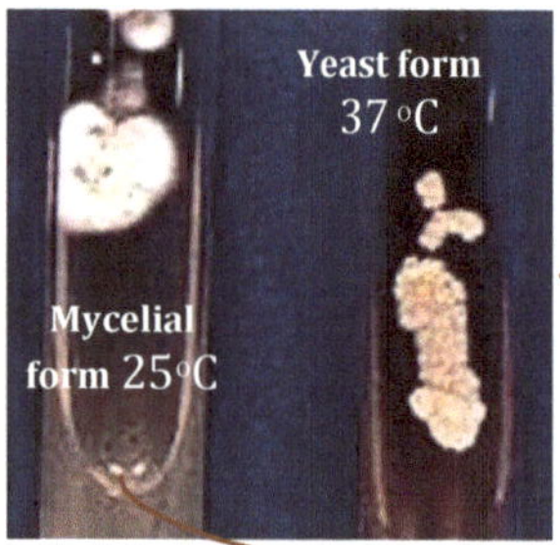

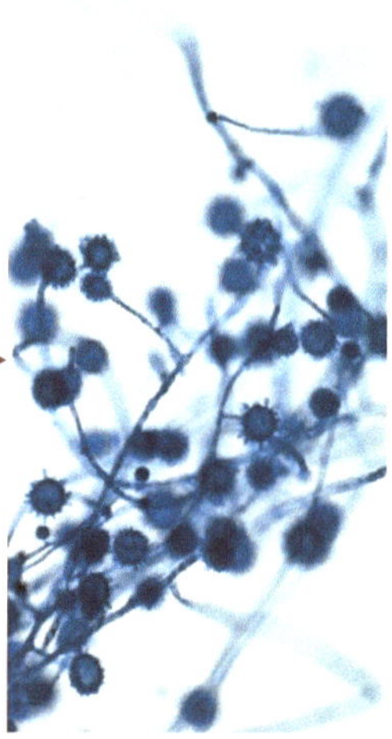

1. *Blastomyces dermatitidis*
2. *Coccidioides immitis*,
3. *Histoplasma capsulatum*,
4. *Paracoccidioides brasiliensis*,
5. *Penicillium marneffei*,
6. *Sporothrix schenckii*,
7. *Ustilago maydis*, also
8. "*Candida albicans* is considered dimorphic"

Fungal growth

- YEASTS
- DEMATIACEOUS MOLDS
- HYALINE MOLDS
- DIMORPHIC FUNGI

Blastomyces dermatitidis, Candida albicans, Coccidioides immitis, *Histoplasma capsulatum*, Paracoccidioides brasiliensis, Penicillium marneffei, Sporothrix schenckii, Ustilago

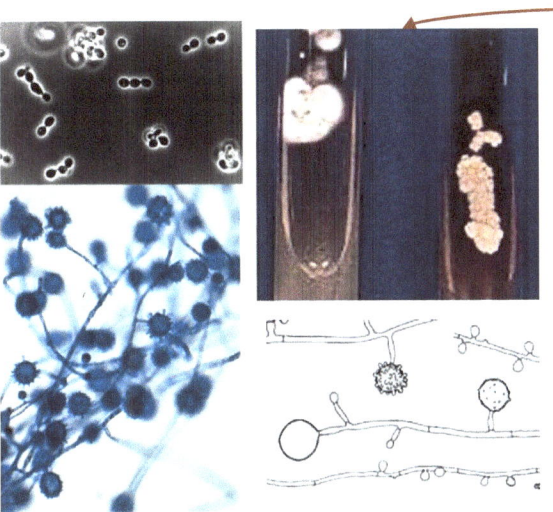

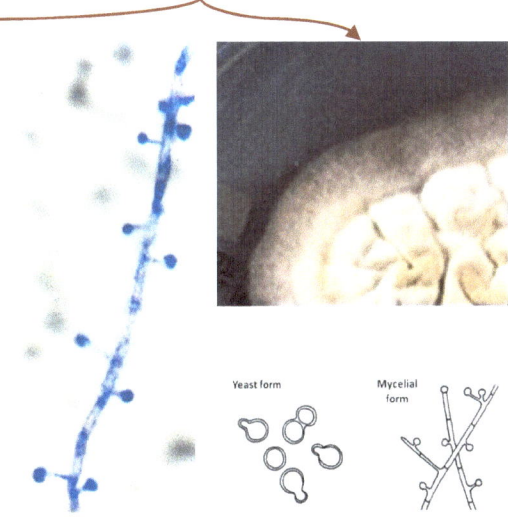

Histoplasma capsulatum

Mycelial form: On SDA at 25C, colonies are slow growing, white or buff-brown, suede-like to cottony with a pale yellow-brown reverse. Other colony types are glabrous or verrucose, and a red pigmented strain has been noted.
Microscopically: morphology shows the presence of characteristic large (8-14 um in diameter), rounded, single-celled, tuberculate macroconidia formed on short, hyaline, undifferentiated conidiophores. Microconidia, if present, are small (2-4 um in diameter), round to pyriform and borne on short branches or directly on the sides of the hyphae.
Yeast form: On brain heart infusion (BHI) blood agar incubated at 37C, colonies are smooth, moist, white and yeast-like. Microscopically: numerous small round to oval budding yeast-like cells, 3-4 x 2-3 um in size are observed

Blastomyces dermatitidis

Mycelial form: On SDA at 25C, colonies are variable in both morphology and rate of growth. They may grow rapidly, producing a fluffy white mycelium, or slowly as glabrous, tan, non-sporulating colonies. Growth and sporulation are enhanced by nitrogenous substances found in starling dung and yeast extract. Most strains become pleomorphic with age. Microscopically, hyaline, ovoid to pyriform, one-celled, smooth-walled conidia (2-10 um in diameter) of the Chrysosporium type, are borne on short lateral or terminal hyphal branches. **Yeast form:** On blood agar at 37C, colonies are wrinkled and folded, glabrous and yeast-like. Microscopically, the organism produces the characteristic yeast phase as seen in tissue pathology

Fungal growth

YEASTS — **DEMATIACEOUS MOLDS** — **HYALINE MOLDS** — **DIMORPHIC FUNGI**

*Blastomyces dermatitidis, Candida albicans, **Coccidioides immitis**, Histoplasma capsulatum, Paracoccidioides brasiliensis, Penicillium marneffei, **Sporothrix schenckii**, Ustilago maydis*

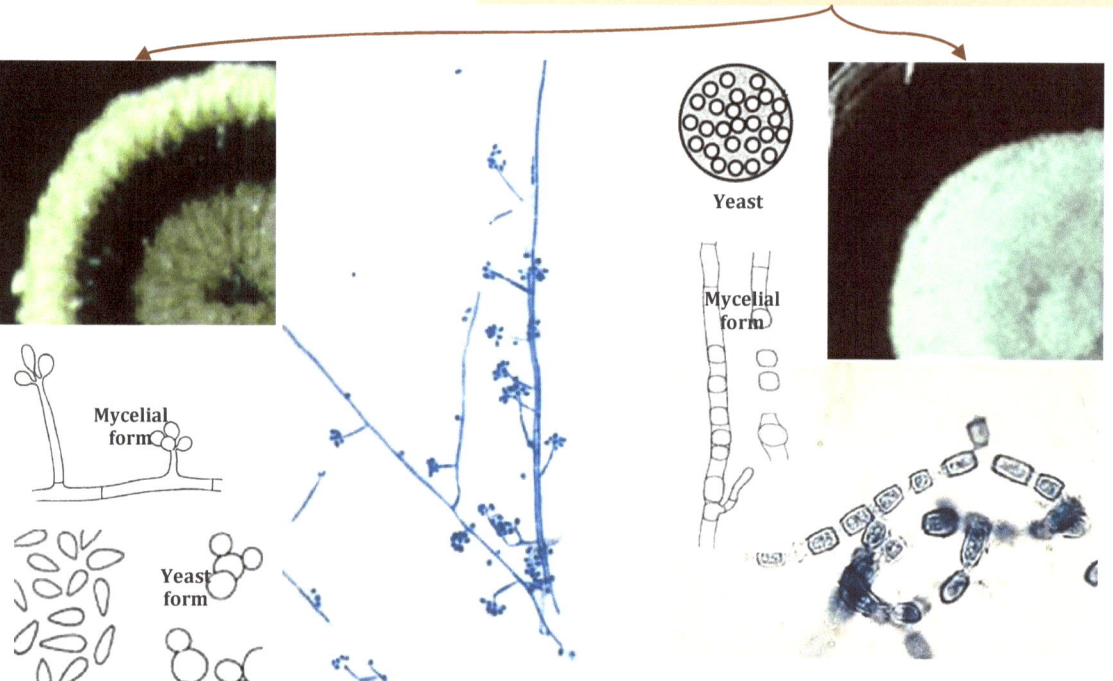

Sporothrix schenckii

At 25C, colonies are slow growing, moist and glabrous, with a wrinkled and folded surface. Some strains may produce short aerial hyphae and pigmentation may vary from white to cream to black. Conidiophores arise at right angles from the thin septate hyphae and are usually solitary, erect and tapered towards the apex. Conidia are formed in clusters on tiny denticles by sympodial proliferation of the conidiophore, their arrangement often suggestive of a flower. As the culture ages, conidia are subsequently formed singly along the sides of both conidiophores and undifferentiated hyphae. Conidia are ovoid or elongated, 3-6 x 2-3 um in size, hyaline, one-celled and smooth-walled. In some isolates, solitary, darkly pigmented, thick-walled, one-celled, obovate to angular conidia may also be observed along the hyphae. On BHI blood agar at 37C, colonies are glabrous, white to greyish yellow and yeast-like, consisting of spherical or oval budding yeast cells

Coccidioides immitis/posadasii complex

Recently Coccidioides immitis has been recognized as 2 species: C. immitis and C. posadasii (Fisher et al. 2002). The two species are morphologically identical and can be distinguished only by genetic analysis and different rates of growth in the presence of high salt concentrations (C. posadasii grows more slowly). C. immitis is geographically limited to California's San Joaquin Valley region, whereas C. posadasii is found in the desert regions of the USA southwest, Mexico and South America. The two species appear to coexist in the desert regions of the USA southwest and Mexico. Colonies of C. immitis/posadasii on Sabouraud's dextrose agar at 25C are initially moist and glabrous, but rapidly become suede-like to downy, greyish white with a tan to brown reverse, however considerable variation in growth rate and culture morphology has been noted. <u>Microscopy</u> shows typical single-celled, hyaline, rectangular to barrel-shaped, alternate arthroconidia, 2.5-4 x 3-6 μm in size, separated from each other by a disjunctor cell. This arthroconidial state has been classified in the genus Malbranchea and is similar to that produced by many non-pathogenic soil fungi, e.g. Gymnoascus species

Fungal growth

- YEASTS
- DEMATIACEOUS MOLDS
- HYALINE MOLDS
- **DIMORPHIC FUNGI**

Blastomyces dermatitidis, **Candida albicans**, *Coccidioides immitis*, *Histoplasma capsulatum*, *Paracoccidioides brasiliensis*, **Penicillium marneffei**, *Sporothrix schenckii*, *Ustilago maydis*

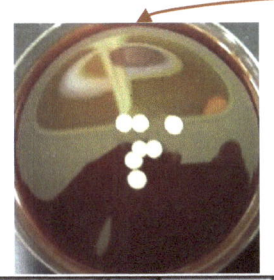

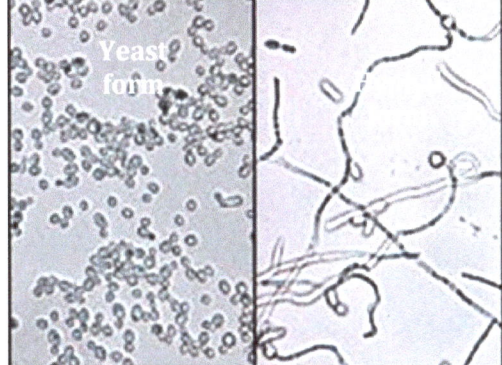

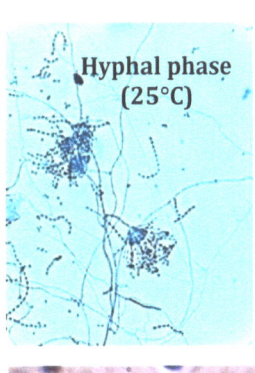

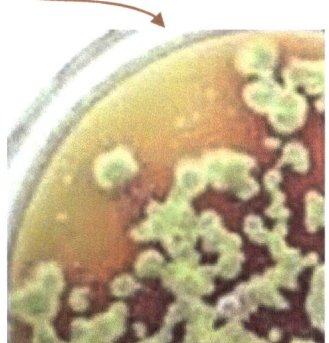

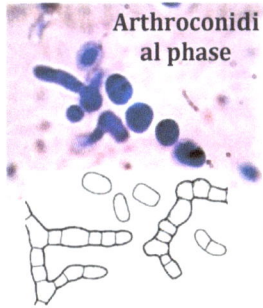

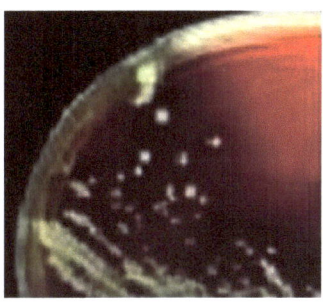

Candida albicans

Candida albicans grows rapidly in culture, reaching maturity in as little as three days. Colonies are cream coloured, raised, entire, smooth & butyrous. On enriched media such as Blood Agar, or Chocolate Agar, the colonies may develop small striations or outgrowths often referred to as "feet" which are indicative of the Candida albicans species. A smear made from colonies taken from Sabouraud-Dextrose Agar, or blood agar will appear as round to oval cells about 4 to 8 μm. Though the cell wall structure differs from that of gram positive bacteria, yeast cells retain the crystal-violet stain of the routine gram stain and therefore appear purple. The yeast cell divides by budding. On primary media (reduced nutritionally) the budding can create elongated cells which when lined up along the dividing plane, mimic the appearance of a hyphae however these inline individual cells are referred to as a pseudohyphae (false hyphae). Some true hyphae may also be formed.
Along side of the pseudohyphae, Candida albicans develops blastoconidia around the area of the 'septa' (division). These appear as smaller round 'grape-like' clusters

Penicillium marneffei

Hyphal phase (37°C): On SDA at 25C, colonies are fast growing, suede-like to downy, white with yellowish-green conidial heads. Colonies become greyish-pink to brown with age and produce a diffusible brownish-red to wine red-pigment. <u>Microscopically:</u> Conidiophores are hyaline, smooth-walled and bear terminal verticils of 3 to 5 metulae, each bearing 3 to 7 phialides. Conidia are globose to subglobose, 2 to 3 um in diameter, smooth-walled and are produced in basipetal succession from the phialides.
Arthroconidial phase (37°C): On brain heart infusion (BHI) blood agar incubated at 37C, colonies are rough, glabrous, tan-colored and yeast-like. <u>Microscopically</u>, yeast-cells are spherical to ellipsoidal, 2 to 6 um in diameter, and divide by fission rather than budding. Numerous short hyphal elements are also present

SECTION FOUR: A SUMMARY TABLE

SPECIMEN COLLECTION, FUNGAL STAINS, CULTURES AND COMMONLY ISOLATED FUNGI FROM DIFFERENT BODY SITES

				Stains		Culture		
Body sites	**Volume**	**Guidelines for collection**	**Storage temp.**	KOH&/or CW	India ink	BHIA + 5% Blood	BHIA+ Blood+ Antibiotic &/or SDA+ Antibiotic	**Commonly isolated agents**
Abscess, wound								
Pus, Exudates, and Drainage	1-5 mL	Using a sterile needle and syringe, aspirate material from un-drained abscesses. Place the material in a sterile container	4°C	Yes	No	No	Yes	*Cryptococcus neoformans Candida* spp., *Sporothrix schenkii, Histoplasma capsulatum, Blastomyces dermatitidis, Coccidioides immitis, Paracoccidioides brasiliensis, Aspergillus* spp., *Phialophoria* sp., *Scedosporium* sp. *(Pseudoallescheria)*
Body fluids								
Blood	20-30 mL (Child 1-5 mL)	Clean the area with disinfectant (70% alcohol, 1-2% iodine) at the time of collection. Use 0.05% sodium polyanethol sulfonate as an anticoagulant [Adults: 20-30 mL; Children: 1-5 mL]. Sent to lab. ASAP (deliver to the lab within 2 hours of collection). Store at 30-37°C if short delay in processing is anticipated. Prepare several smears for Giemsa, Gram and PAS staining. Culture the remaining specimen [remaining 3-5 ml of marrow and blood may be cultured on the media]. Inoculate 0.5-1.0 ml of buffy coat of blood, prepared by centrifuging 5-10 ml of blood, onto the surface of the media	30-37°C	Yes	No	Yes	No	*Candida albicans, Aspergillus* spp., [endocarditis]
Bone marrow	3-5 mL	Aspirate 3-5 ml of bone marrow and place it in a sterile container. 0.05% sodium polyanethol sulfonate or heparin as an anticoagulant can be added. The pediatric isolater blood culture system may be used.	30-37°C	Yes	No	Yes	No	

Summary Table continued ...

Body sites	Volume	Guidelines for collection	Storage temp.	Stains		Culture		Commonly isolated agents
				KOH &/or CW	India ink	BHIA + 5% Blood	BHIA+ Blood+ Antibiotic &/or SDA+ Antibiotic	
Bones and joints								
Needle aspiration, Arthrocentesis	2 mL	Sterile preparation of site, collected by physician in sterile screw capped or snap cap tubes. Handle as a STAT (immediately) specimen and transport immediately	4°C	Optional	No	Yes	No	*Candida albicans, Aspergillus* spp., *Cry. neoformans, Blastomyces dermatitidis, C. immitis* [osteomyelitis]; *Sporothrix schenkii, Coccidioides immitis, Candida albicans* [arthritis]
Central Nervous System [meningitis/encephalitis]								
CSF	2 mL	Sterile preparation of site, collected by physician in sterile screw capped or snap cap tubes. Obtain 4-5 mL of CSF for optimal recovery. Handle as a STAT (immediately) specimen and transport immediately. Do not refrigerate	30-37°C	No	Yes	Yes [+ BHIB]	No	*Cryptococcus neoformans, Histoplasma capsulatum, Coccidioides immitis, Candida albicans*
Brain abscess aspirate	2 mL	Sterile preparation of site, collected by physician in sterile screw capped or snap cap tubes. Obtain 4-5 mL of CSF for optimal recovery. Handle as a STAT (immediately) specimen and transport immediately	4°C	No	Yes	Yes [+ BHIB]	No	*Cryptococcus neoformans, Candida* spp., *Coccidioides immitis, Aspergillus* spp.
Ear [otitis externa]								
Swab [outer canal]	Swab or few discharge drops	Clean the skin around the ear with a mild antiseptic. Moisten a swab in sterile saline and roll around ear canal in a circular manner. Insert the swab into a sterile screw-cap tube containing the appropriate transport media [as for bacteria]	4°C	Yes	No	No	Yes	*Aspergillus* spp., *Candida albicans*
Eye								
Corneal scraping	Scraping / swab	Notify the lab before beginning the procedure. Media will be provided by laboratory to be inoculated at the bedside. Small swab from each eye or Corneal scraping (by physician). For keratitis, ophthalmologist scrape the surface of the cornea, usually in a surgical procedure	4°C	Yes	No	No	Yes	*Fusarium solani, Aspergillus* spp., *Candida* spp.

Summary Table continued ...

Body sites	Volume	Guidelines for collection	Storage temp.	Stains		Culture		Commonly isolated agents
				KOH &/or CW	India ink	BHIA + 5% Blood	BHIA+ Blood+ Antibiotic &/or SDA+ Antibiotic	
Conjunctival discharge/ swab	Swab or few discharge drops	Clean skin around the eye with a mild antiseptic. Moisten a swab in sterile saline and roll over the conjunctiva. Insert the swab into a sterile screw-cap tube containing the appropriate transport media	4°C	Yes	No	No	Yes	*Candida albicans, Candida* spp. *Sporothrix schenkii, Aspergillus* spp., *Histoplasma capsulatum*
Gastro-intestinal tract (peritonitis, visceral abscess)								
Stool	2 gm or a rectal swab	Pass stool directly into a large leak proof container. Or use the stick provided	4°C	Optional	No	Yes	No	*Candida albicans, Aspergillus* spp., *Fusarium* spp.
Peritoneal fluid	50 mL	Disinfect the skin with iodine tincture. Specimens are obtained via needles aspiration or surgery. Transfer to sterile container or blood culture bottles	4°C	No	No	Yes	No	*Candida albicans, Aspergillus* spp., *Fusarium* spp.
Genital tract								
Genital ulcer swab	Swab	Using several sterile swabs, collect material from the vagina. Insert swabs into a sterile tube	4°C	Optional	No	No	Yes	*Histoplasma capsulatum*
Vaginal swab/ discharge	1-5 mL/ swab	Using several sterile swabs, collect material from the vagina. Insert swabs into a sterile tube	4°C	Optional	No	No	Yes	*Candida albicans, Candida* spp.
Granulomatous infections								
Aspirate, exudates	1-5 mL/	Submit in sterile container without formalin Specimen may be kept moist with 0.85% sterile saline.	4°C	Optional	No	No	Yes	*Cryptococcus neoformans, Candida* spp., *Sporothrix schenkii, Histoplasma capsulatum,*
Biopsy	1 cc tissue	Tissue is aseptically collected from the center and edge of the lesion Place between moist gauze squares, add a small amount of sterile water or 0.85% NaCl to keep tissue from drying out, and Send to the laboratory	4°C	Optional	No	No	Yes	*Blastomyces dermatitidis, Coccidioides immitis, Paracoccidioides brasiliensis, Aspergillus* spp., *Phialophoria* sp., *Scedosporium* sp. *(Pseudoallescheria)*
Respiratory tract, upper/ mouth								
Oral/throat swab [thrush]	Swab	Using sterile swabs, collect material from throat inflamed area. Insert swabs into a sterile tube or use transport media	4°C	Optional	No	No	Yes	*Candida albicans*

Summary Table continued .....

Body sites	Volume	Guidelines for collection	Storage temp.	Stains		Culture		Commonly isolated agents
				KOH &/or CW	India ink	BHIA + 5% Blood	BHIA+ Blood+ Antibiotic &/or SDA+ Antibiotic	
Sinus aspirate [allergic sinusitis]	1-3 mL	Sterile preparation of the site collected by physician in sterile screw capped or snap cap tubes. Handle as a STAT (immediately) specimen and transport immediately	4ºC	Optional	No	No	Yes [+ BHIB]	*Aspergillus* spp.
Respiratory tract, lower								
Sputum	2-10 mL	Collect the first morning specimen Have patient rinse mouth and collect sputum resulting from a deep cough, or if necessary by induction Have patient expectorate immediately into a sputum collection container. Do not let patient hold sputum in the mouth place cap on conical centrifuge tube, tighten, label, and transport to the laboratory Discard remaining pieces of the collection device at the patient's bedside	4ºC	Optional	Optional	No	Yes	*Pneumocystis carinii, Cryptococcus neoformans, Histoplasma capsulatum, Blastomyces dermatitidis, Coccidioides immitis, Paracoccidioides brasiliensis, Aspergillus* spp., *Phycomyces* spp.
Bronchial washings, bronchial lavage, lung biopsies, and tracheal aspirates	2 mL	These specimens are collected aseptically by the physician, placed in the appropriate container and immediately transported to the lab	4ºC	Optional	Optional	No	Yes	
Pleural, Thoraoce-ntesis	2 mL	These specimens are collected aseptically by the physician, placed in the appropriate container and immediately transported to the lab	4ºC	Optional	No	Yes	No	*Candida albicans, Aspergillus* spp., *Fusarium* sp.

Summary Table continued ...

Body sites	Volume	Guidelines for collection	Storage temp.	Stains			Culture	Commonly isolated agents
				KOH &/or CW	India ink	BHIA + 5% Blood	BHIA+ Blood+ Antibiotic &/or SDA+ Antibiotic	
Skin								
Hair	11 hair	Select infected areas and with forceps, epilate at least 10 hairs. For hairs broken off at the scalp level, use a scalpel or a blade knife. Place hairs between two clean glass slides or in a clean envelope labeled with the patient's data.	RT	Yes	No	No	Yes [+DTM)]	*Dermatophytes [Trichophyton, Microsporum, Epidermophyton* spp.] *Candida albicans, Malassezia furfur, Trichosporon beigelii, Candida albicans*
Nails	Cut nails or scraping	Clean the nail with 70% alcohol. Dorsal plate - Scrape outer surface and discard; scrape the deeper portion. Remove a portion of debris from under the nail with a scalpel. Collect whole nail or nail clippings. Place all material in a clean envelope labeled with the patient's data.	RT	Yes	No	No	Yes [+DTM]	
Scrapings	Scraping	Wipe lesions and interspaces with alcohol sponge or sterile water. Scrape the entire lesion(s) and both sides of interspaces with a sterile scalpel. Place scrapings between two clean glass slides or place in a clean envelope labeled with the patient's data	RT	Yes	No	No	Yes [+DTM]	
Tissue [soft]								
Subcutaneous tissue biopsy, exudates, grains	1 cc tissue	Tissue is aseptically collected from the center and edge of the lesion. Place between moist gauze squares, add a small amount of sterile water or 0.85% NaCl to keep tissue from drying out, and Send immediately to the laboratory	4°C	Optional	No	No	Yes	Mycetoma agents [*Madurella* sp., *Cladosporium* sp.], *Candida albicans, Aspergillus* spp., *Blastomyces dermatitidis Sporothrix schenkii,* Zygomycetes [*Rhizopus* spp., *Mucor* spp.]
Urinary tract [cystitis pyelonephritis],								
Urine	>20 mL	Early morning specimens are aseptically collected in sterile containers	4°C for up to 12-14 hrs	Optional	Optional	No	Yes	*Candida albicans, Candida* spp., *Cryptococcus neoformans*

BHIA = Brain heart Infusion agar; BHIB = Brain heart Infusion broth; SDA= Sabouraud's Dextrose Agar; DTM = Dermatophyte test medium; CW = Calcofluor White

Section Five: Culture media, Stains and Microscopic techniques

Culture media

Sabouraud Dextrose Agar (SDA)

Description

SDA is a selective medium for the cultivation of pathogenic and nonpathogenic fungi, particularly dermatophytes, and yeasts. The acidic pH (5.6) of the medium inhibits many species of bacteria.

Diagnostic Features

Structures such as spores and pigmentation are well developed on this medium.

Composition

Dextrose 40g; Peptone mixture 10g; Bacteriological Agar 15; DW 1L; Final pH 5.6.

Preparation

- Suspend/dissolve 65 g powder (Difco) in 1 L of DW or purified water
- Mix thoroughly
- Heat the contents with frequent agitation and boil for 1 minute to completely dissolve the powder
- Avoid overheating which could cause a softer medium
- Autoclave at 121°C for 15 minutes
- Test samples of the finished product for performance using stable, typical control cultures

Microorganisms Growth

Aspergillus niger ATCC 16404	good to excellent
Candida albicans ATCC 26790	good to excellent
Escherichia coli ATCC 25922	good to excellent
Lactobacillus casei ATCC 9595	good to excellent
Saccharomyces cerevisiae ATCC 9763	good to excellent

Sabouraud Dextrose Agar with antibiotics

Composition

Dextrose 40g, Peptone mixture 10g, Cycloheximide (Actidione) 0.4g, Chloramphenicol 0.05g, Bacteriological Agar 15g, DW 1L; Final pH 5.6.

Preparation

- Suspend/dissolve 65 g powder (Difco) in 1L of DW or purified water
- Mix thoroughly
- Heat the agar media with frequent agitation and boil for 1 minute to completely dissolve the powder

- Avoid overheating which could cause a softer medium
- Autoclave at 121°C for 15 minutes
- Aseptically add 0.4g cyclohexamide and 0.05g Chloramphenicol to each liter of autoclaved, cooled medium (at 55°C)
- Test samples of the finished product for performance using stable, typical control cultures

MICROORGANISMS GROWTH:

Candida albicans	Good growth
Trichophyton mentagrophytes	Good growth
Candida tropicalis	partially inhibited
Penicillium spp.	partially inhibited
Cryptococcus neoformans	partially inhibited
Aspergillus fumigatus	partially inhibited
Scedosporium (Pseudoallescheria)	partially inhibited
Escherichia coli	partially inhibited

BRAIN HEART INFUSION BROTH (BHIB)

DESCRIPTION

BHI Broth is a nutritious, buffered culture medium that contains infusions of brain and heart tissue and peptones to supply protein and other nutrients necessary to support the growth of fastidious and non-fastidious microorganisms.

COMPOSITION

Ingredients (Grams/Liter): Calf brains (infusion from 200g) 12.5; Beef heart (infusion from 250g) 5.0; Proteose peptone 10.0; Sodium chloride 5.0; D(+)-Glucose 2.0; Disodium hydrogen phosphate 2.5; DW 1L. Final pH 7.4. Store dehydrated powder, in a dry place, in tightly-sealed containers at 2-25°C.

PREPARATION

- Suspend 37 g powder in 1 L DW
- Mix thoroughly
- Heat with frequent agitation and boil for 1 minute to completely dissolve the powder
- Autoclave at 121°C for 15 minutes
- Cool to 50°C, mix well and distribute into tubes, plates or flasks
- Store prepared media below 8°C, protected from direct light

Brain Heart Infusion Agar (BHIA) with 5% Sheep Blood

BHI agar is a nutritious, buffered culture medium that contains infusions of brain and heart tissue and peptones to supply protein and other nutrients necessary to support the growth of fastidious and non-fastidious microorganisms. Blood is added to this medium to enhance growth of fastidious fungi such as *Histoplasma capsulatum*.

Composition

Ingredients (Grams/Liter): Calf brains (infusion from 200g) 12.5; Beef heart (infusion from 250g) 5.0; Proteose peptone 10.0; Sodium chloride 5.0; D(+)-Glucose 2.0; Disodium hydrogen phosphate 2.5; Agar 10.0; Final pH 7.4. Store dehydrated powder, in a dry place, in tightly-sealed containers at 2-25°C.

Preparation

- Suspend 47 g in 950 mL of distilled water
- Boil to dissolve the medium completely
- Sterilize by autoclaving at 121°C for 15 minutes
- Cool to 50oC, aseptically add 50 ml defibrinated blood, mix well
- Distribute into tubes, plates or flasks
- Store prepared media below 8°C, protected from direct light.

BHIA with 5% Sheep Blood and antibiotics

Composition

Ingredients (Grams/Liter): Calf brains (infusion from 200g) 12.5; Beef heart (infusion from 250g) 5.0; Proteose peptone 10.0; Sodium chloride 5.0; D(+)-Glucose 2.0; Disodium hydrogen phosphate 2.5; Agar 10.0; Final pH 7.4 +/- 0.2 at 37°C. Store dehydrated powder, in a dry place, in tightly-sealed containers at 2-25°C. Antibiotic solution can be added: e,g, 0.05 gram chloramphenicol and 0.05 gram gentamicin +/- cyclohexamide (0.5gram). Or Streptomycin 0.04gm + Penicillin 20000 U +/- cyclohexamide (0.5gram)

Preparation

- Suspend 47 g in 950 mL of distilled water
- Boil to dissolve the medium completely
- Sterilize by autoclaving at 121°C for 15 minutes
- Cool to 50oC, aseptically add 50 ml defibrinated blood, mix well
- Distribute into tubes, plates or flasks
- Store prepared media below 8°C, protected from direct light.

Dermatophyte Test Medium (DTM)

Description

DTM is a selective and differential medium used for the detection and presumptive identification of dermatophytes from clinical specimens.

Composition

Papaic Digest of Soybean Meal 10.0 g, Dextrose 10.0 g, Phenol Red 0.2 g, Cycloheximide 0.5 g, Agar 20.0 g, DW 1L.

Preparation

- Suspend 40.5 g of the powder in 1 L of purified water.
- Mix thoroughly.
- Heat with frequent agitation and boil for 1 minute to completely dissolve the powder
- Autoclave at 121°C for 15 minutes
- Cool to 50°C and add gentamicin sulfate and chloramphenicol (0.1 g of each per L)
- Test samples of the finished product for performance using stable, typical control cultures.

STAINS

10% POTASSIUM HYDROXIDE (KOH)

USE

For the direct microscopic examination of skin scrapings, hairs, nails and other clinical specimens to see fungal elements.

PREPARATION

Dissolve 10g KOH in 90 mL water, mix and then add 10 mL glycerol, mix gently. 20% KOH are also used, it can be prepared by dissolving 20g KOH in 90 mL water, mix and then add 10 mL glycerol, mix gently.

MAKING MOUNTS FOR MICROSCOPY

- Using an inoculation needle remove a small portion of the specimen, especially from any necrotic or purulent areas, and mount in a drop of KOH on a clean microscope slide
- Cover with a coverslip, squash the preparation with the gentle pressure
- Blot off the excess fluid
- Gently heat by passing through a flame two or three times. Do not boil
- Wait 20 minutes for skin scrapings to several hours for nail scrapings (specimen cleared)
- Examine microscopically for the presence of "refracting" fungal elements

Note: negative specimens should be kept and re-examined the next day to avoid reporting false negative results due to delayed clearance and staining of the specimen

10% POTASSIUM HYDROXIDE (KOH) WITH PARKER INK

USE

This stain is same as 10% KOH but addition of parker ink enhances visibility of fungal elements. For the direct microscopic examination of skin scrapings, hairs, nails and other clinical specimens to see fungal elements.

PREPARATION

Dissolve 10g KOH in 80 mL water, mix and then add 10 mL glycerol and 10 mL Parker ink permanent blue ink then mix gently.

MAKING MOUNTS FOR MICROSCOPY

- Using an inoculation needle remove a small portion of the specimen, especially from any necrotic or purulent areas, and mount in a drop of KOH on a clean microscope slide
- Cover with a coverslip, squash the preparation with the gentle pressure
- Blot off the excess fluid
- Gently heat by passing through a flame two or three times. Do not boil
- Wait 20 minutes for skin scrapings to several hours for nail scrapings (specimen cleared)

- Examine microscopically for the presence of faintly blue stained fungal elements

Note: negative specimens should be kept and re-examined the next day to avoid reporting false negative results due to delayed clearance and staining of the specimen.

Lactophenol Cotton Blue (LPCB)

Use

For the staining and microscopic identification of fungi from cultures.

Composition

Cotton Blue (Aniline Blue) 0.05 g ; Phenol Crystals ($C_6H_5O_4$) 20 g ; Glycerol 40 mL; Lactic acid ($CH_3CHOHCOOH$) 20 mL; Distilled water 20 mL.

This stain is prepared over two days:
- On the first day, dissolve the Cotton Blue in the distilled water. Leave overnight to eliminate insoluble dye
- On the second day, wearing gloves add the phenol crystals to the lactic acid in a glass beaker. Place on magnetic stirrer until the phenol is dissolved
- Add the glycerol
- Filter the Cotton Blue and distilled water solution into the phenol/glycerol/lactic acid solution
- Mix and store at room temperature

India ink

Use

To demonstrate the capsule which is seen as an unstained halo around the organisms distributed in a black background. This is employed for fungal diagnostics especially for *Cryptococcus neoformans*.

Composition

Black charcoal ash (pulverize); Distilled water, Glycerol or gelatin; vinegar

Homemade preparation of India ink:
- Place the charcoal ash in the small bowl
- Add water slowly and stir with the hard bristled brush it the charcoal dissolved
- Add few drops of vinegar and mix thoroughly to create stability in the ink once it has dried
- Place the ink in a tight lid jar
- Ink is now ready to use

Staining Procedure

- Place a loopful of India ink on the side of a clean slide
- A small portion of the solid culture is suspended in saline on the slide near the ink and then emulsify in the drop of ink, or else, mix a loopful of liquid culture of specimens like CSF with the ink

- Place a clean cover slip over the preparation avoiding air bubbles
- Press down, or blot gently with a filter paper strip to get a thin, even film
- Examine under dry objectives followed by oil immersion

CALCOFLUOR WHITE WITH 10% KOH

USE

Direct microscopic examination of skin scrapings, hairs, nails and other clinical specimens to see fungal elements. Calcofluor white (M2R powder from Polysciences) or Blankophor BA (from Bayer) are used as whitening agents by the paper industry and selectively bind to cellulose and chitin. The dye fluoresces as it is exposed to ultraviolet light. This as a very sensitive method, however, a fluorescence microscope with the correct ultraviolet filters is required.

PROCEDURE

Solution A Potassium hydroxide reagent.
- Dissolve the KOH in water and add glycerol.
- Potassium hydroxide 10 g
- Glycerin 10 ml
- Distilled water 90 ml

Solution B Calcofluor white reagent.
- Dissolve Calcofluor white powder in the distilled water by gentle heating.
- Calcofluor white 0.1 g
- Distilled water 100 ml

METHOD FOR MAKING MICROSCOPIC MOUNTS

Mix one drop of each solution on the centre of a clean microscope slide.

Place the specimen in the solution and cover with a coverslip, squash the preparation with the butt of the inoculation needle and then blot off the excess fluid.

Gently heat the slide and examine microscopically for the presence of fungal elements that fluoresce a chalk-white or brilliant apple green color, depending on the filters used.

Comments: This is a very rapid and sensitive method; however a fluorescence microscope fitted with filters to give an excitation with ultraviolet light below 400 nm wavelength is required.

Gram's stain

Use

Detection of Gram positive and gram negative bacteria as well as yeast elements in tissue and smears from cultures. This is an essential stain and should be used whenever bacteria or yeasts is suspected.

Method

– Saturate a dry fixed smear with crystal violet for 1 min, then Rinse with water

– Saturate the smear with iodine for 1 min, Rinse again

– Decolorize with Gram decolorizes (acetone/alcohol) for 20 seconds, and Rinse

– Counter stain with safranin for 1 min, Rinse

– Carefully blot the slide dry with bibulous paper and Observe under the microscope. Gram + stain purple; Gram - stain red/pink.

– Negative specimen should be kept and re-examine next day

Grocott's Methenamine Silver (GMS) stain

Use

Detection of fungal elements in tissue sections. This is an essential stain and should be used whenever a fungal etiology is suspected.

Mechanism

Chromic acid treated fungi possess aldehydes which will reduce the hexamine-silver mixture to produce a black deposit, i.e. an argentaffin reaction. Fungi stain black.

Solutions

- 5% aqueous chromic acid
- 1% aqueous sodium bisulphite
- 5% aqueous borax
- 0.1% aqueous gold chloride
- 2% aqueous sodium thiosulphate

Stock Methenamine Silver solution

    Add 5 ml of 5% silver nitrate to 100 ml of 3% hexamine. A white precipitate will form which, on shaking, will dissolve. This solution will keep from 1-2 months at 4°C.

Working silver solution (filter before use)

    Stock methenamine silver solution 25 ml

    Distilled water 25 ml

    5% Borax 1-2 ml

Method

- Take sections to water (transfer)

- Oxidize in 5% chromic acid for 1 hour.
- Wash in running tap water for 10 minutes.
- Treat with sodium bisulphite for 1 minute to remove any residual chromic acid.
- Wash in tap water then distilled water.
- Place section in the working silver solution at 60°C in a water bath.
- Rinse in distilled water.
- Tone in 0.1% gold chloride for 5 minutes.
- Rinse in distilled water.
- Remove unreduced silver by treating with 2% sodium thiosulphate for 1-2 minutes
- Wash thoroughly.
- Counterstain with Light green.
- Dehydrate clear and mount in D.P.X.

Safety Precautions

Silver nitrate is toxic and skin contact should be avoided; methenamine is a flammable solid and an irritant; chromic acid is also toxic. Therefore, when preparing any of the above solutions protective clothing should be worn, including gloves, aprons and protective glasses. Any spill should be mopped up immediately with water.

Periodic acid-Schiff (PAS)

Use

For the demonstration of glycogen and neutral mucins. Useful for the detection of fungal elements in tissue sections.

Mechanism

Certain tissue elements are oxidized by periodic acid to produce aldehydes. These aldehydes will react with Schiff's reagent to produce a magenta colored compound. In the PAS Digest, the glycogen is digested by salivary amylase present in saliva.

Solutions

1% Periodic acid (50% vol.)

- Periodic acid 2 ml
- Distilled water 98 ml

Schiff's reagent:

- Basic Fuchsin (C.I. 42500) 1 g
- Potassium metabisulphite 2 g
- Distilled water 200 ml
- HCl concentrate 2 ml
- Deactivated Charcoal 1-2 g

Boil distilled water, add basic fuchsin slowly, mix and cool to 50°C. Add potassium metabisulphite. Mix and cool to room temperature before adding HCl. Keep in the dark overnight for bleaching to occur. Add charcoal and filter through coarse filter paper, then fine filter paper. Store in fridge

METHOD

- Take sections to water (transfer)
- Treat with 1% periodic acid for 5 minutes
- Rinse in water.
- Treat with Schiff's reagent for 10 minutes.
- Wash in running tap water for 5 minutes (this develops the color).
- Counterstain nuclei lightly with Mayer's Hematoxylin for 1 minute.
- Wash and "blue up" in Li2Co3.
- Dehydrate, clear and mount in D.P.X.

Results: PAS positive material - magenta; Nuclei - blue; PAS digest material – colorless

GIEMSA'S STAIN

PRINCIPLE AND USE

Giemsa stain is used to differentiate nuclear and/or cytoplasmic morphology of platelets, RBCs, WBCs, and parasites

COMPOSITION

Stock solution

- Dissolve 3.8g of Giemsa powder into 250ml of methanol
- Heat the solution from step 1 to ~60oC
- Slowly add in 250ml of glycerin to the solution from step 2
- Filter the solution from step 3
- The solution needs to stand a period of time prior to use. Although times vary based on who you ask a minimum of two months is usually recommended

Working solution

- Add 10ml of stock solution to 80ml of distilled water and 10ml of methanol

PROCEDURE

- Place a clean 1- by 3-in. glass microscope slide on a horizontal surface.
- Place a drop (30 to 40 µL) of blood onto one end of the slide about 0.5 in. from the end
- Using an applicator stick lying across the glass slide and keeping the applicator in contact with the blood and glass, rotate (do not "roll") the stick in a circular motion while moving the stick down the glass slide to the opposite end.
- The appearance of the blood smear should be alternate thick and thin areas of blood that cover the entire slide.
- Immediately place the film over some small print and be sure that the print is just.

Microscopic techniques

Tease mount technique

Use

A simple method for the rapid mounting of sporulating fungi. It may damage some structures and loose important features for identification.

Method

- Wear gloves and work in a BSC
- Pick small portion of colony with its underlying agar using a dissecting needle
- Place it on a drop of Lactophenol Cotton Blue(LPCB)
- on a clean slide [*placed slide on top of an inverted Petri dish*]
- Tease gently the colony apart with the dissecting needle
- Overlay [cover] with coverslip
- Apply gentle pressure using the eraser of a pencil to make an even mount
- Examine fungal elements with 10X then 40X then 100X
- **Advantage:** *Easy to use*
- **Disadvantage:** *Disturbs the delicate fruiting fungal structure and spores*

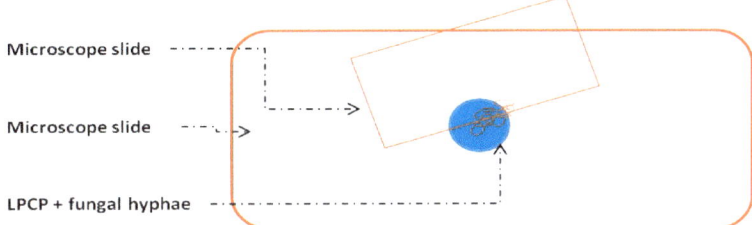

Cellotape Flag Preparations

Use

An excellent technique for the rapid mounting of sporulating fungi because it keeps more of the reproductive structures intact.

Method

- Using clear 2 cm wide cellotape and a wooden applicator stick (orange stick) make a small cellotape flag (2x2cm)
- Using sterile technique, gently press the sticky side of the flag onto the surface of the culture

- Remove and apply a drop of 95% alcohol to the flag, this acts as a wetting agent and also dissolves the adhesive glue holding the flag to the applicator stick
- Place the flag onto a small drop of LPCB on a clean glass slide, remove the applicator stick and discard, add another drop of stain, cover with a cover slip, gently press and mop up any excess stain

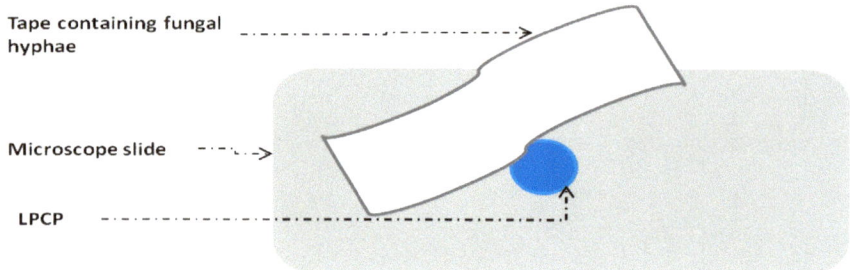

MICRO CULTURE (SLIDE CULTURE) TECHNIQUE

USE

To observe the precise arrangement of the conidiophores and the way in which spores are produced (conidial ontogeny) be studied virtually in situ with as little disturbance as possible

METHODS

One plate of nutrient agar; potato dextrose is recommended, however, some fastidious fungi may require harsher media to induce sporulation like cornmeal agar or Czapek dox agar

Using a sterile blade cut out an agar block (7 x 7 mm) small enough to fit under a coverslip

Flip the block up onto the surface of the agar plate

Inoculate the four sides of the agar block with spores or mycelial fragments of the fungus to be grown

Place a flamed coverslip centrally upon the agar block

Incubate the plate at 26C until growth and sporulation have occurred

Remove the cover slip from the agar block

Apply a drop of 95% alcohol as a wetting agent

Gently lower the coverslip onto a small drop of Lactophenol cotton blue on a clean glass slide

The slide can be left overnight to dry and later sealed with fingernail polish

When sealing with nail polish use a coat of clear polish followed by one coat of red colored polish

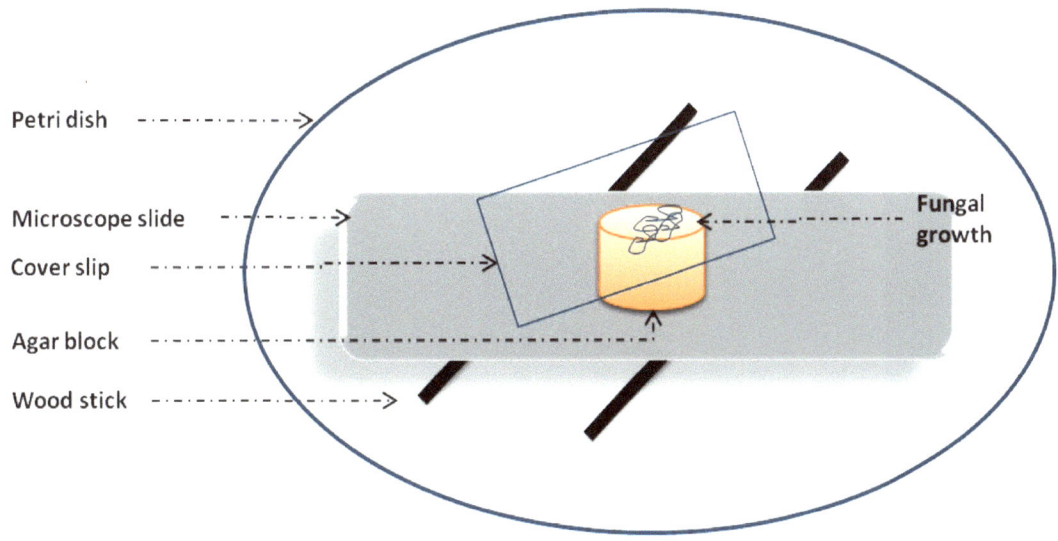

REFERENCES

1. Koneman's Color Atlas and Textbook of Diagnostic Microbiology (Color Atlas & Textbook of Diagnostic Microbiology). Elmer W. Koneman Lippincott Williams & Wilkins; 6th Edition (2005)

2. Bailey & Scott's Diagnostic Microbiology, 12th Edition, By B.A. Forbes et al., (2007)

3. Medically Important Fungi: A Guide to Identification. By Larone DH, 3rd ed. ASM Press, Washington, D.C. 1995

4. Mycology Online, The University of Adelaide, David Ellis, School of Molecular & Biomedical Science, The University of Adelaide, AUSTRALIA 5005 (http://www.mycology.adelaide.edu.au/) Accessed Feb, 2012

5. Doctor Fungus, Doctor Fungus (http://doctorfungus.org/) http://website.nbm-mnb.ca/mycologywebpages

6. World of Dermatophytes: A pictorial (http://www.provlab.ab.ca/mycol/tutorials/derm/dermwho.htm)

7. Mycobank: Fungal databases (http://www.mycobank.org/DefaultPage.aspx)

8. La Mycologie sur le Web (http://coproweb.free.fr/mycoweb/indexmyc.htm)

INDEX

A

A. pullulans, 37
Abscess, 59
Absidia, 41, 42, 43
Acidic pH, 65
Acremonium, 47, 48, 49, 50, 52, 53
Actidione, 65
Agar, 63, 65, 67, 68
Algae, 8
Allergies, 9
Alternaria, 35, 36, 37, 38, 39
Amanita mushroom, 9
Ameroconidia, 49
Anthrophilic, 45
Antibiotic solution, 67
Apophysate, 41
Apophysomyces elegans, 42
Arthroconidi, 57
Arthroconidia, 31, 32, 33, 34, 37, 45, 56
Arthroconidial phase (37°C), 57
Aseptate hyaline hyphae, 40, 41, 42, 43, 44, 45, 46, 47, 48, 49, 50, 52, 53
Asexual, 8
Aspergillosis, 18
Aspergillus, 5, 9, 59, 60, 61, 62, 63, 65, 66
Aspergillus flavus, 51
Aspergillus fumigatus, 51
Aspergillus nidulans, 51
Aspergillus niger, 51
Aspergillus sp, 11, 14, 16
Aspergillus spp., 23, 25, 26
Aspergillus terreus, 51
Aspirate, exudates, 61
Aureobasidium, 37

B

B. dermatitidis, 17
B. ranarum, 43
Basidiobolus, 18, 43
Beauvaria bassiana, 47
Beauveria, 47, 48, 49, 50, 52, 53
Beta-lactam antibiotics, 9
BHI, 66, 67
BHI blood agar, 37
BHIA + Blood, 15, 23, 24, 25, 26, 27, 28, 29
Biohazard bag, 12
Biopsy, 61
Bipolaris, 35, 36, 37, 38, 39
Black bread molds, 40
Black charcoal ash, 70
Blacked grained eumycotic mycetoma, 11, 20
Blastoconidia, 32, 33, 34
Blastomyces, 23, 47, 48, 49, 50, 52, 53, 54, 55, 56, 59, 61, 62, 63
Blastomyces dermatitidis, 55, 59, 61, 62, 63
Blastomycosis, 17
Blastoschizomyces, 32, 34
Bleach, 12
Blood, 12, 25, 59, 60, 61, 62, 63, 67
Body fluids, 59
Bone marrow, 12, 25, 59
Brain abscess, 26
Brain heart infusion (BHI), 55, 57
Bronchial lavage, 62
Bronchial washings, 62
Brown sclerotic bodies, 20
BSC, 12, 75
Budding, 8

C

C. coronatus, 43
C. immitis, 56
C. posadasii, 56
Calcofluor white, 11, 71
Calcofluor White, 63, 71
Candida 5, 11, 25, 27, 28, 29, 32, 33, 34, 54, 55, 56, 59, 60, 61, 62, 65, 66,
Candida albicans, 11, 25, 27, 28, 29, 33, 54, 55, 56, 57, 59, 63
Candida dubliniensis, 33
Candida spp 59, 60, 61, 63
Candida spp., 28, 29, 32, 33, 34
Candidiasis, 19, 28
Cellotape Flag Preparations, 75
Chaetomium, 35, 36, 37, 38, 39
Charcoal ash, 70
Chemoheterotrophic, 8
Chitin, 8, 71
Chlamydoconidia, 44
Chromoblastomycosis, 20
Chrysosporium, 47, 55
Cladophialophora, 35, 36, 37, 38, 39
Cladosporium, 24, 27, 35, 36, 37, 38, 39, 63
Clinical specimens, 11
Coccidioides immitis, 19, 26, 28, 54, 56, 59, 60, 61, 62
Coccidioidomycosis, 19
Columellae, 41, 42
Conidia in chains, 35, 47, 48, 49, 50, 52, 53
Conidia in singles or, 35, 36, 37, 38, 39
Conidiobolus, 43
Conidiophores, 36, 39, 43, 44, 48, 49, 50, 53, 55, 56, 77
Conjunctival discharge/swab, 60
Corneal, 11
Cryptococcosis, 17
Cryptococcus, 11, 14, 16, 17, 23, 26, 27, 32, 33, 34, 59, 60, 61, 62, 63, 66, 70
Cryptococcus neoformans, 11, 14, 16, 17, 23, 26, 27, 32, 59, 60, 61, 62, 63, 66, 70
CSF, 11, 12, 14, 15, 16, 26, 60, 71
Culture, 11, 15
Culture media, 64, 65
Cunninghamella, 42
Curvularia, 35, 36, 37, 38, 39
CW, 11, 28, 59, 60, 61, 62, 63
Cycloheximide, 65, 68
Cystitis, 63
Cysts, 19

D

Decomposers, 8
Dematiaceous, 8
Dematiaceous (pigmented) molds, 8
Dematiaceous molds, 32, 35, 36, 37, 38, 39
Dermatological, 11, 12, 14, 15, 16
Dermatological specimens, 12
Dermatophyte Test Medium, 68
Dermatophytes, 5, 11, 15, 22, 25, 26, 28, 65, 68
Dermatophytes, 22, 63, 78
Dermatophytosis, 22
Dextrose, 31, 63, 65, 68
Digestion of skin sample, 14, 16, 22
Dimorphi c fungi, 32
Dimorphic fungi, 8
Direct microscopy, 11, 14, 16
Disinfectant, 13, 59
Drainage, 27
Drechslera, 35, 36, 37, 38, 39
DTM, 3, 15, 22, 63, 68

E

Ecosystems, 8

Epicoccum, 35, 36, 37, 38, 39
Epidermophyton, 22, 44, 45, 46, 63
Exophiala, 20, 35, 36, 37, 38, 39
Exophiala jeanselmei, 20
Exserohilum, 35, 36, 37, 38, 39
Exudates, 27
Exudates, and drainage, 59
ETT, 23

F

F. oxysporum, 52
Fonsecaea, 35, 36, 37, 38, 39
Fragmentation, 8
Fugal growth, 31, 32, 33, 34, 35, 36, 37, 38, 39, 40, 41, 42, 43, 44, 45, 46, 47, 48, 49, 50, 52, 53, 54, 55, 56
Fungal hyphae, 18
Fungi, 2, 3, 5, 6, 8, 9, 15, 20, 22, 23, 25, 26, 27, 28, 29, 31, 36, 40, 49, 54, 59, 65, 67, 70, 72, 75, 77
Fungus, 5, 8, 15, 48, 77
Fusarium, 47, 48, 49, 50, 52, 53, 60, 61, 62
Fusarium solani, 60

G

Genital ulcer swab, 61
Geotrichum, 32, 33, 34
Geotrichum penicillatum, 34
Giemsa, 4, 17, 25, 59, 74
Giemsa's stain, 17, 74
Gliocladium, 47, 48, 49, 50, 53
GMS, 3, 11, 17, 18, 19, 72
Gomori methamine, 17
Grains, 27
Gram's stain, 72
Grocott's Methenamine Silver, 72

H

H & E, 11, 17, 18, 20
Haematoxylin and Eosin, 17
Hair, 14, 15, 16, 22, 45, 63
Histopathology, 11, 17
Histoplasma, 11, 15, 17, 23, 26, 28, 47, 48, 49, 50, 52, 53, 54, 55, 56, 59, 60, 61, 62, 67
Histoplasma capsulatum, 11, 15, 17, 23, 26, 28, 48, 54, 55, 56, 57, 59, 60, 61, 62, 67

Histoplasmosis, 17
Household bleach, 12
Hyaline, 18, 31, 34, 36, 37, 40, 43, 44, 48, 49, 50, 52, 53, 55, 56
Hyaline hyphomycetes, 40, 41, 42, 43, 44, 45, 46, 47, 48, 49, 50, 52, 53
Hyaline molds, 8, 32, 40, 41, 42, 43
Hyphae, 8
Hyphal phase (25°C), 57

I

IMA, 15, 23, 24, 25, 26, 27, 28, 29
India ink, 3, 11, 14, 16, 26, 29, 59, 60, 61, 62, 63, 70, 71
Indirect microscopy, 11

K

KOH, 11, 22, 59, 60, 61, 62, 63, 69, 71
KOH wet mount, 11

L

Lactophenol Cotton Blue, 11, 70, 75, 77
Lichens, 8
Lipophilic, 33
LPCB, 4, 11, 22, 28, 70, 75, 76

M

Macroconidia, 44, 45, 46, 48, 55
Madurella, 11, 20, 24, 27, 47, 48, 49, 50, 52, 53, 63
Malassezia furfur, 19, 22, 33, 63
Micro culture, 77
Microconidia, 44, 45, 52
Microsporum, 22, 44, 45, 46, 63
Mildew, 9
Mold form, 37
Mold hyphae, 14, 16
Molds, 8, 9, 22, 23, 24, 25, 26, 27, 28, 31, 35, 47, 48
Mortierella, 41
Mould form of *Blastomyces*, 47
Moulds, 8, 14, 16
Mounts, 69, 71
Mucor pusilluss, 18
Mucor sp., 18
Mucor spp., 63
Muriform, 35, 36, 37, 38, 39
Mycetoma, 63

Mycetoma (actinomycetoma), 20
Mycetoma (eumycotic), 20
Mycocladus, 41, 42
Mycocladus corymbifera, 41
Mycology, 8, 78
Mycorrhizae, 8
Mycosel agar, 15

N

Nails, 14, 15, 16, 22, 45, 63, 69, 71
Non septate hyphae, 31
Non-inhibitory media, 15, 22, 23, 24, 25, 26, 27, 28, 29

O

Otitis externa, 60

P

P. marneffei, 17, 49
Paecilomyces, 47, 48, 49, 50, 52, 53
Paracoccidioides brasiliensis, 54, 56, 57, 59, 61, 62
Parker Ink, 69
PAS stain, 17, 19, 59, 73, 74
Penicilliosis, 17
Penicillium, 9, 49, 53, 54, 56, 66
Penicillium chrysogenum, 49
Penicillium marneffei, 49, 54, 56, 57
Peptone, 65
Periodic acid-Schiff, 17, 73
Peritoneal fluid, 61
Peritonitis, 61
Phaeohyphomycosis, 20
Phialides, 36, 49, 50, 52, 53
Phialophora, 35, 36, 37, 38, 39, 59, 61
Phoma, 35, 36, 37, 38, 39
Phycomyces spp., 62
Pithomyces, 39
Pneumocystis carinii, 62
Pneumocystis jiroveci, 19
Pneumocystis pneumonia, 19
Poisonous, 9
Potassium hydroxide, 69
Presence of budding yeast cells, 17
Presence of grains, 20
Presence of hyphae, 18
Presence of pseudohyphae and yeast cells, 19
Presence of sclero tic bodies, 20

Presence of spherules, 19
Pseudoallescheria, 59, 61, 66
Pseudohyphae, 19, 28, 31, 32, 33, 34
Pus, 27, 59
Pycnidia, 35, 36, 37, 38, 39
Pyelonephritis, 63

R

R. atrovirens, 37
R. schulzeri, 37
Ramichoridium, 37
Rejection of clinical specimens, 13
Respiratory specimens, 23
Rhinocladiella, 35, 37
Rhinosporidiosis, 19
Rhinosporidium seeberi, 19
Rhizoids, 41, 42
Rhizopus, 24, 27, 41, 42, 43, 63
Rhizopus oryzae, 41
Rhizopus spp., 24, 27, 32, 33, 34, 63
Ringworm, 22
Rusts, 9

S

S. schenkii, 37
Sabouraud Dextrose Agar, 32, 57, 65
Saccharomyces cerevisiae, 65
Saksenaea, 41, 43
Saksenaea vasiformis, 41
Saprophytic fungi, 12
Scedosporium, 47, 59, 61, 66
Scedosporium apiospermum, 47
Scopulariopsis, 49
Scrapings, 14, 15, 22, 63, 69, 70, 71
SDA, 3, 15, 22, 31, 32, 35, 40, 45, 47, 48, 49, 50, 52, 53, 55, 59, 60, 61, 62, 63, 65
SDABH, 15, 22, 23, 24, 25, 26, 27, 28, 29
Sepedonium sp., 48

Septate hyaline hyphae, 40, 41, 42, 43, 44, 45, 46, 47, 48, 49, 50, 52, 53
Septate hyphal elements, 31
Septate, branching fungal hyphae, 11
Sexual reproduction, 43
Single yeast cells, 31, 32
Skin, 11, 14, 16, 19, 22, 60, 61, 69, 70, 71, 73
Slide Culture, 77
Slow growing, 35
Smuts, 9
Sodium hypochlorite, 12
Spills, 12
Sporangia, 19, 41, 42
Sporangiophores, 41, 42
Sporothricosis, 17
Sporothrix, 17, 24, 27, 36, 37, 38, 39, 54, 56, 59, 60, 61, 63
Sporothrix schenkii, 24, 27, 57, 59, 60, 61, 63
Sporulation, 8, 41, 47, 53, 55, 77
Sputum, 23, 62
Stemphylium, 35, 36, 37, 38, 39
Sterols, 8
Stool, 61
Subcutaneous nodule, 20
Subcutaneous tissue, 63
Symbiosis, 8
Syncephalastrum, 41, 42

T

Tease mount technique, 75
Tinea, 19, 22, 46
Tinea versicolor, 19
Tissue, 11, 17, 18, 19, 20, 22, 23, 24, 48, 61, 63, 66, 67, 72, 73
Tissue [soft], 63
Tissue biopsy, 24
Torulopsis, 32
Trans+ longitudinal divided (Muriform)conidia, 35
Transversely-divided conidia, 35, 36, 37, 38, 39
Trich. mentagrophyte, 45

Trich. soudanense, 45
Trich. terrestre, 45
Trich. tonsurans, 45
Trich. verrucosum, 45
Trichoderma, 47, 48, 49, 50, 52, 53
Trichophyton, 15, 22, 44, 45, 46, 63, 66
Trichophyton sp., 15
Trichosporon beigelii, 34, 63
Trichosporon spp., 34
Trichosporonosis, 19

U

Ulocladium, 35, 36, 37, 38, 39
Urine, 29, 63
Ustilago maydis, 54, 57

V

Vaginal discharge, 28
Vaginal swab, 28
Vaginal swab/ discharge, 61
Vaginal thrush, 28
Verticillium, 53

W

Wangiella dermatitidis, 20
Wound, 59

Y

Yeast cells with capsules, 14, 16
Yeast form, 11, 17
Yeastlike cells, 20
Yeasts, 8, 17, 19, 22, 23, 24, 25, 26, 27, 28, 32, 33, 65, 72

Z

Zoophilic, 45
Zygomycetes, 40, 41, 42, 43, 44, 45, 49, 50, 52, 53, 63
Zygomycosis, 18
zygophores, 43
Zygospores, 8, 43

www.ingramcontent.com/pod-product-compliance
Lightning Source LLC
Chambersburg PA
CBHW050738180526
45159CB00003B/1268